'This is a brilliant resource. The ic
the educational components of th
therapeutic space for students to e
allow children to enjoy the schoo
teachers with a means to unlock th

*– Sylvia Simonyi-Elmer, Ph. ... psychotherapist, certified sandplay therapist and senior teacher-supervisor, Kingston, Ontario*

'This is one of the most exciting and moving educational books I have read in the past 20 years. It emerges out of considerable reflection and hands-on teaching with a wide range of children. The writer takes a developmental perspective that builds on profound symbolic and affective experiences which lead to major advances in the cognitive and social domains. Her approach combines the wisdom of the past with the latest findings from the neurosciences. The methods and suggestions outlined in the book guarantee both excitement and success for pupils and teachers alike. I recommend this book most highly.'

*– John Allan, Ph.D., Professor Emeritus, Education, University of British Columbia, Vancouver and author of* Inscapes of the Child's World: Jungian Counselling in Schools and Clinics

'In her book *Sandtray Play and Storymaking: A Hands-On Approach to Build Academic, Social, and Emotional Skills in Mainstream and Special Education,* Sheila Dorothy Smith issues an invitation to all of us who work with children, especially teachers. She gently challenges us to think outside the box and use what is natural, joy-creating, meaning-making and fun – play, stories and symbols – to develop happier, calmer, more receptive and self-disciplined children. Her approach is evidence based, well researched, practical and useful. It makes sense and it works. Try it and you may even have some fun, too!'

*– Mary Shirley-Thompson, M.A., Manager of Services, Children's Mental Health, Family, Youth and Child Services of Muskoka*

'*Sandtray Play and Storymaking* is remarkable! In the book, Sheila demonstrates the extraordinary results that can be achieved through the inclusion of psychological insight in education. Her method of creating, telling and recording sandtray worlds and stories gives children a means to express their inner thoughts and feelings, allows teachers to gain a better understanding of their students and provides the perfect platform for developing literacy skills.'

*– Dr Allan Guggenbühl, psychologist, educationalist and Jungian analyst, University of Education of the State of Zurich*

'*Sandtray Play and Storymaking* is an exquisite book. It is a beautiful portrayal of this therapeutic modality where children, at play in their classrooms with their sandtrays and figurines, construct their own world – making stories filled with ideas, dreams and realities. During this process, a child's feelings and memories can emerge, blending fantasy and life experience.

Shadows of Sylvia Ashton-Warner, Tolkien, Bettelheim and Jung drift through the narrative alongside the children's written versions of their creations, encouraging readers to find their own sandtrays and begin again.'

*– David Booth, Professor Emeritus, OISE, University of Toronto*

Sheila Dorothy Smith

# Sandtray Play and Storymaking

## A Hands-On Approach to Build Academic, Social, and Emotional Skills in Mainstream and Special Education

Jessica Kingsley *Publishers*
London and Philadelphia

Figure 2.2 on p.35 from *Growing Up Again* by Jean Illsey and Connie Dawson, 1998 is reprinted with permission from Hazelden Publishing.
Permissions for case studies, photographs, writing and interview comments was kindly granted by the families and guardians of the children featured in this book.

First published in 2012
by Jessica Kingsley Publishers
116 Pentonville Road
London N1 9JB, UK
and
400 Market Street, Suite 400
Philadelphia, PA 19106, USA

*www.jkp.com*



**Library of Congress Cataloging in Publication Data**
Smith, Sheila Dorothy.
Sandtray play and storymaking : a hands-on approach to build academic, social, and emotional skills in mainstream and special education / Sheila Dorothy Smith.
p. cm.
Includes bibliographical references.
ISBN 978-1-84905-205-4 (alk. paper)
1. Teaching--Aids and devices. 2. Sandboxes. 3. Creative teaching. 4. Affective education. 5. Problem children--Education. I. Title.
LB1044.88.S65 2012
371.33--dc23
2012002879

**British Library Cataloguing in Publication Data**
A CIP catalogue record for this book is available from the British Library

ISBN 978 1 84905 205 4
eISBN 978 0 85700 436 9

Printed and bound in Great Britain

*For Georgia Eleanor Grainger*
*in memory of her great-grandmother*
*Dorothy Ethelwyn Thomas*

# CONTENTS

# ACKNOWLEDGEMENTS

On the walls of the foyer of Huntsville Public School is a wide-spreading tree. Painted there by a mother in the community, the tree speaks of the welcome and shelter that the school offers to children and also to ideas such as those chronicled here. For the support, participation, and enthusiasm of the parents, teaching staff, and administrators of this school, I am deeply grateful. Special thanks to those teachers who shared the stories from their classrooms – Jane Keevil, Christopher Kemp, and Cheryl Schmid. And, to Andrea Slocombe, who conferred with me in the heady early days often until the sun set and the classroom darkened, my heartfelt gratitude for the ongoing contributions of her wide expertise, generous insight, and kindred understanding.

A number of people deserve special acknowledgement for assistance provided during the research and writing of this book. David Booth first told me that this was a book and guided me through the process of bringing it to completion with unflagging good cheer. Brendan Harding provided thoughtful early reading of the manuscript and steady encouragement. My daughter Rachel Smith and her husband Brett Grainger gave clear-sighted direction and skilled editorial assistance along with discussions over tea and laughter. Thanks go as well to Trillium Lakelands District School Board, Eusebia Da Silva, Linda Duvall, Kim Goodwin-Myers, Tina Gute Bowering, Liz Hollands, Maria Iosue, Denise Jordan, John Loewy, Vicky Mathies, Wendy Nicholson, Florence Riley, Jennifer and Peter Smith, Duff Smith, Valerie Stam, Barb Willms, and Brenda Weinberg. Finally, glad thanks to my husband Glen, my long companion in the building, telling, and listening of our life together.

# PREFACE

This book first began in a special education classroom where 12 students, defiant and disengaged, began to build worlds in the sand and to tell and write the stories of those worlds. I watched as the storymaking that sprang from hands-on imagination sparked the students' engagement in learning the language arts of speaking, listening, and narrative writing. I have here attempted not only to supply you with a map for recreating these techniques in your own contexts, but to theorize some of what I saw happen, drawing on multiple sources in order to better understand what unfolded before my eyes in a way that was initially so seemingly miraculous. The book contains multiple genres: it is a chronicle, a manual, and a work of theory. But at root it is an encounter with children who have breathed into its pages the immediacy and power of their sandworlds and their stories. For their lively, direct, ongoing teaching, I thank them, over and over again.

Chapter 1

# ROOTS

*'It's like we have been looking for treasure our whole lives and what is buried in our mind has come through.'*

– Devlin, Grade 6 (age 11)

One afternoon, the second last of the school year, five Grade 6 (age 11) boys knocked at the door of the special education resource room. They had a surprise for me – a movie, filmed as a series of testimonials about sandtray play. The movie is accompanied by the startling visual images of their sandworlds and by the sound of Hedley, a Canadian band, singing about how over and over again, and in no time at all, boys grow up into men. The words of the script are unrehearsed and spontaneous:

*You just have what's in your mind out there.*
*You get to explore places.*
*Thanks for letting me explore with my imagination.*
*It is a lot of fun.*
*We get to make stories with sand creations.*
*I wouldn't change it.*
*We create new ideas while we play.*
*I had better friends.*
*We get this opportunity to explore our minds.*
*We get a lot of choice.*
*Each week we create different worlds. They become the settings for our stories.*
*I love exploring through my ideas.*
*All it takes is a good brain and a bucket of sand!*
*We get to play with ideas with a whole world.*
*We are really thankful.*

> *You get to spread your imagination so far, just like the planes are going to go really far across the country.*
> *Where we got to go had treasure.*
> *My favourite part is that we get to explain it to the whole group. And after that you get questions and appreciations.*
> *We love hanging out with our friends and exploring our ideas.*
> *It has been a real adventure.*
> *Where you get to explore places.*
> *It's like we have been looking for treasure our whole lives and what is buried in our mind has come through.*
> *We...we just say thank you now.*

'Intelligence,' writes Simone Weil, 'functions only in joy. Intelligence is perhaps even the only one of our faculties to which joy is indispensable. The absence of joy asphyxiates it' (1987, p.123). These boys are reporting on joy: 'explore', 'explore through', 'create', 'make', 'spread far', 'have fun', 'have choice', 'play', 'love'. The activities of play are one and the same as the activities of thought and imagination: *You just have what's in your mind out there.*

## HOW IT ALL BEGAN

It was mid-November about three and a half years earlier. We were five educators – teacher, special education teacher, administrators, consultant – meeting around a table in the special education resource room. Stark late-autumn sunlight shone through the windows, giving the air a sharp-edged clarity that contrasted with the woolly perplexity that we were feeling. It was two months into the school year, many meetings into the process, and we were stumped. The matter at hand was one cohort of seven- to nine-year-olds.

'There are too many students who are struggling, too few who can act as role models,' the vice-principal eventually offered flatly.

This was a possible definition of the problem. The class lacked the critical mass of students who could act as role models and mentors for those who needed it. There were too many students with severely disruptive behaviours, too few with school-adjusted behaviours. The balance was off. Gavin, huddled inside his sweatshirt hood, rebuke in his hunched shoulders; Abel, whose 'This is *stupid*' punctuated the day, and Darius whose reflexes were finely tuned to react to Abel's opinions; Darcie whose silence was a fortress; Morty who, unable to use words clearly, spoke in tantrums; Lucy, who, on days when she did come to school, lingered at her coat hook, sobbing: these were some of the citizens of that small world. They traded with each other in the currency of the put-down. Sullenness had seeped in and settled like a grey fog.

This cohort had a history together, a culture that had been formed since kindergarten. Their current classroom teacher – a versatile, compassionate veteran – had doggedly attempted everything in the learning strategies tool kit: individual and class contracts, check marks and stars, individual education plans, privileges withdrawn, privileges awarded, the 'problem-solving room', 'marbles in a jar', class meetings, class celebrations, behaviour logs, meetings with parents, responsive seating arrangements. All these strategies had been tried. But still something needed to change. The culture of this class – the air they breathed, the soil in which they were rooted – needed to change.

## Breathing out

There was something freeing about this November meeting: the freedom that comes out of acknowledgement of failure and a dearth of solutions, born of permission to think outside the box. The day after the meeting, a phrase of Sylvia Ashton-Warner, a teacher of Maori children in the 1950s, nudged my memory: 'It's [the child's] native right to breathe normally' (1980, p.250).

'Breathe normally.' The phrase reminded me of a different class in a different school, years earlier, where I had first encountered Ashton-Warner's writing. A friend and colleague, Kirsty Williamson, had introduced me to the book *Teacher* (1963), when I confessed to my frustration that, after four years of teaching kindergarten, the work was no longer satisfying, the classroom without vitality. The fact is that I had been taken hostage by my own anxiety about performance: *Would my students be prepared academically for Grade 1 (age six)? Would they reach the letter and sight word recognition targets, print awareness, phonological awareness expectations?* The worry over my students' end-of-year achievements had cast a long shadow, reconfiguring the classroom as a struggle. I had at first adopted the stance of cheerleader, a stance that was shifting incrementally towards bossiness. The fact is that neither cheerleader nor drill sergeant are postures conducive to the 'I and thou' of the teacher/learner bond. No wonder the class had lost its spirit, the five-year-olds becoming unruly.

Ashton-Warner understood that attention needed to be paid to the irreducible fact that each child is a whole world of thought and feeling. Each brings daily into the classroom her unique experience, knowledge, and needs. For the teacher, acknowledging that fact and honouring it is the starting point. Children need to express before they can receive; they need to breathe out the inner life – their hopes and fears and the reality in which they live and bring with them to the schoolroom – before they can breathe in the skills and knowledge the schoolroom wishes to impart. Ashton-Warner devised for her classroom a daily rhythm of 'output' and 'intake': student-selected, expressive activity, in which children create, followed by teacher-directed activity in which they receive new information. 'What's so unusual in arranging, in allowing...a child's day into spans of output and intake? It's only breathing. Deep breathing of the mind,' she writes. 'It's [the child's] native right to breathe normally' (1980, p.249). A rhythm like the tides is contained in her words.

Reading *Teacher*, I had the feeling of coming home, of recognizing what I had known all along but had forgotten. I decided to invite the children to 'breathe out' as Ashton-Warner described, in an effort to bring the classroom back from a field of contest to a garden – a '*kinder-garten*'. At the beginning of each day, the children were given time to play in the fundamental substances of clay, sand, and water before they were called to meet for instruction. Group sharing and teacher input waited until the students had individual opportunity to create. The children gave expression to their own reality, their own stories, before they were given new information to absorb.

It worked. The class regained its sense of equilibrium and vitality. And, not surprisingly, the students mastered the required skills for Grade 1 (age six).

Many years later, following the problem-solving team meeting of that November morning, the memory of the shift in that long-ago kindergarten returned to me as the intimation of a possible solution. Maybe, I thought, the same invitation to 'breathe normally' needs to be issued to this group of students in this late autumn of their school year. The team agreed.

It was decided that for 90 minutes each day I would work with the 12 seven- and eight-year-olds who comprised the younger half of the class, using the rhythm of output followed by input. The children's own stories, discovered through play and expressed during the output segment, would be the material with which they would work in order to develop literacy skills.

## THE PLAN IN A NUTSHELL: BUILD, TELL, LISTEN, RECORD

The 'breathing out' would happen through play. The child psychotherapist Garry Landreth observes: 'Toys are used by children like words and play is their language' (1993, p.17). To access their own stories, the students needed to speak the universal language of children. They needed to play. Given that opportunity, they would discover their ideas.

Individual sandtrays and miniature figures that were replicas of everything in the physical and mythical world would be the equipment provided.

In a classroom adaptation of the therapeutic modality of sandplay, the students would build a world in the sand, tell the story of that world, listen to their peers' stories, and record their own in writing. The worlds the children would make in their trays and the stories they told about them would emerge out of the storehouse of their creativity. The sand would engage both hands and imagination. The plan would be the 'light enough touch' that Ashton-Warner describes:

> What a dangerous activity teaching is. All this plastering on of foreign stuff. Why plaster on at all when there is so much inside already? So much locked in? If only I could get it out and use it as working material. And not draw it out either. If I had a light enough touch it would just come out under its own volcanic power. (1963, p.14)

Sandtray play – unworded, hands-on, active imagination – would lend its energy to the pedagogical goals of the language curriculum, the worded activities of speaking, listening, and writing. Enlisting this kind of play in the service of language learning would be in keeping with Dewey's perspective that 'teachers must start with the experience and interests of students and patiently forge connections between that experience and whatever subject matter was prescribed' (as cited in Noddings 1992, p.19). The workshop would be structured as follows:

- *Building:* The students would build a world in their individual sandtrays using the miniatures provided to them.
- *Telling and listening:* After building, the students would tell the story of their sandworld to a listening partner. The children would learn how to organize and sequence the telling of their own narratives and how to listen and respond respectfully as their classmates shared their stories.
- *Recording:* In order to preserve their stories after they created them orally, the students would learn the craft of writing. It would be their own stories that would provide both the impetus and the working material for this learning.

On the first Monday of December, the experiment began. Day by day, students built self-contained worlds that expressed a story. Each student heard and responded to a partner's story and practised the skills of attentive listening. Entrance and exit to the classroom were marked by a handshake and individual message to the teacher. Music calmed the atmosphere as the students built worlds, and songs summoned them to group meetings. Students listened and responded to the reading of classic tales and myths. Celebrations marked the days when stories of the sandtray worlds were read to a wider audience. Self-expression, the polite entrance and exit, respectful attention to the child's inner world, the use of play as the child's work, and a sense of belonging for each student all worked together to create a new culture that was characterized by a climate of civility and a sense of community. The dynamic of the classroom began to change. The ecosystem of relation within the collective shifted towards a new balance.

This book is the attempt to unpack what took place and continues to take place out of that beginning. But I am getting ahead with the story. So that you will understand the roots of sandtray play as it was reinterpreted in the school setting, let me ask you to consider first the function and role of play, symbol, and symbol play.

## PLAY AS THE GATEWAY TO THE STORY WITHIN

A child at play is not self-conscious. He is in it with both feet and whole heart, finding delight. Writing about the work of the artist Madeleine L'Engle (1980) helps us understand the activity of play. She notes the distinction between two Greek conceptions of time – *kairos* and *chronos*. Chronos, she observes, is clock-watching time, in which we think about what has happened in the past and what we are going to do next. Kairos is that time which breaks through the chronological. It is present tense. Play belongs to kairos: 'The artist at work is in kairos,' L'Engle writes. 'The child at play, totally thrown outside himself in the game be it building a sand castle or making a daisy chain, is in kairos. In kairos we become what we are called to be as human beings' (1980, p.98).

Play invites in us a kind of concentration and a focus that makes us forget the rest of the world, the small particulars, the quotidian. We look up and cannot believe that so much time has elapsed. Paintings and poetry are artifacts brought back to the daily round from one at play. Created outside of ordinary time, they become what we cherish; they are what help us remember significance, they are entranceways to the space between thoughts. In his classic work, *Homo Ludens*, Huizinga argues that language, myth, and ritual all have their origins in the spirit of play (1955, p.4).

Research-based evidence documents the benefits of play in the child's acquisition of language, social skills, and general development.[1] For a moment, think of a child at play: a boy or a girl, say five or seven

1 See, for example, research presented to the Princeton 2005 symposium on play in Singer, D.G., Golinkoff, R.M., and Hirsh-Pasek, K. (eds) (2006) *Play = Learning: How Play Motivates and Enhances Children's Cognitive and Social-Emotional Growth.* Oxford: Oxford University Press.

or 11 years old. Watch them. Listen. What do you see? What do you hear?

- *Say you are the queen and I am the guard.* The child is exploring conflicting points of view and experimenting with relationships by trying on different roles.
- *You cheated! You can't do that.* For this alternate play world to survive and be viable, the citizens must adhere to its laws. Ignoring the rules shatters the world. That there are rules cannot be in question. The player has only two choices: she must renegotiate the rules or take the consequence of breaking them, which is exclusion. Subservient to the structure and rules of the play, the child is developing an ethical sense.
- *Oh no! The boat has tipped! Help! Sharks!* The child is creating and then solving problems, much in the same way as does the author of a good yarn.
- *I know! Say Leo is our father and he came and he had a rope!* He is creating satisfying resolutions, abandoning unsatisfying ones, and controlling outcomes. He develops a heightened sense of mastery because in play he and his playmates are in control of what transpires.
- *Say the beach towel is my wedding veil.* Play allows experience through imagination, a highly creative process. Children speak whole play worlds into being with the word 'Say' – that 'Say' evocative of Genesis: 'And God said, Let there be light and there was light.'
- *Listen to the laughter.* The child is having fun. Play is fun. It is serious in much the same way that work is serious, but it is also fun. Fun is the irreducible element.
- *Oh no! Can't we stay out for 15 more minutes?* Notice their reluctance when, as the light fades, you summon them from an afternoon of play to the supper table. Immersed and suspended within the time of their alternate world, children at play are learning to extend and sustain attention.

- *Take the witch away!* Joan Bodger (2000) shares an incident reported by Frobenius in which a five-year-old, given three matches to keep her occupied, named them Hansel, Gretel, and Witch. Shortly after beginning to play with them in this way, the child was shrieking, 'Take the witch away!' (p.324). Through her imagination and her active play, the child links story with feelings.

## Understanding symbol

The word symbol comes from the Greek 'sym' and 'ballein' – to throw together. The distinction between metaphor and symbol is a matter for discussion, but it is clear that we are all conversant with using one thing to stand for another and, by so doing, increasing our capacity to communicate. We all use metaphorical and symbolic language in our everyday speech ('I have hit a brick wall', 'She's over the moon', 'He is a snake in the grass'). A hard-to-express inner experience is communicated in quick shorthand through our connecting it with something in the outer world. This is the language of poetry. When, for example, Mary Oliver writes, 'When it's over I want to say all my life / I was a bride married to amazement' (1992, p.10), her words identify an inner feeling, often difficult to express (the desire to be yoked to a sense of wonder) with an outer reality (the bride on her wedding day). Ruminating on Shakespeare's lines, 'The lunatic, the lover and the poet / Are of imagination all compact', Northrop Frye once quipped that all three – lover, lunatic, poet – are the only people who can take metaphor seriously because lovers, lunatics, and poets say two things are the same that are not the same; they state that one thing *is* another (Personal lecture notes, November 10, 1970). Perhaps we are all lovers, lunatics, or poets, because we all do speak in metaphor. Every time we identify one thing with something else, we are speaking that language.

## Symbol play in the sand

In sandplay, symbol and metaphor are communicated with the language of real objects that can be seen, felt, shaped, handled, and touched. The Moon, the Snake, the Brick Wall, the Witch, the Honeybee, the Superhero, the Dragon – each can be placed in the tray or molded in the sand, making possible an expression of the player's inner world. The child of Frobenius' story, if given such tools, might place a witch in the sand and, by so doing, externalize and express her fears. The witch frightens her, and the witch is also a symbol of what is frightening to her.

In sandtray play, the child shapes the terrain of the sand and places within it figurines chosen from an array of objects that are miniature replicas of everything in the real world and the world of fantasy. In the three-dimensional world of the sandtray, experience, event, memory, and emotion can be shown, sorted out, and communicated. Feelings that may be too confusing, overwhelming, or unacceptable to apprehend consciously – let alone to organize – can be given a voice in the space, a voice that speaks in a cryptic pictorial language.

Finding in the outer world an image that is analogous to and in proportion with what we are experiencing in our inner world is freeing, because the feeling does not any more contain us; we contain and dialogue with the feeling. We are no longer flooded with what we cannot name. Often we feel in our bodies the sense of release that this brings.[2] Carl Jung reflects in his memoirs: 'To the extent that I managed to translate the emotions into images – that is to say, to find the images that were concealed in the emotions – I was inwardly calmed and reassured' (1965, p.177).

Although words often accompany the play as dialogue, explanation, or storytelling, there is no necessity for them. The player often gets in touch with a deep impulse, a fundamental feeling. There may be no conscious reason and no known name for what miniature is chosen or why it feels satisfying to place it in the tray. The world is satisfying on a non-verbal level. I recall one summer afternoon when my mother at age 90, engrossed in making a sandtray world, paused for a moment, looked up from it, and said to me, 'I don't know if I am making this or if it is making itself.' In his poem, 'A Prayer for Old Age', Yeats decries

2 Interestingly, recent neurobiological research reported by Holmes confirms that the limbic system of the brain is modulated by 'turning raw feelings into symbols' (as cited in Schore 2000, p.39).

the kind of thinking and thought processes that originate from in the 'mind alone'. By contrast, he writes, 'He that sings a lasting song, / Thinks in a marrow-bone' (1996, p.282).

Sandworlds come from the marrow-bone.

An example of the use of symbol, expressed in different modalities, is seen here in the work of one sandplayer. Here we see cave and light symbols embodied in the sandtray in Figure 1.1, and articulated in the imagery of a poem.

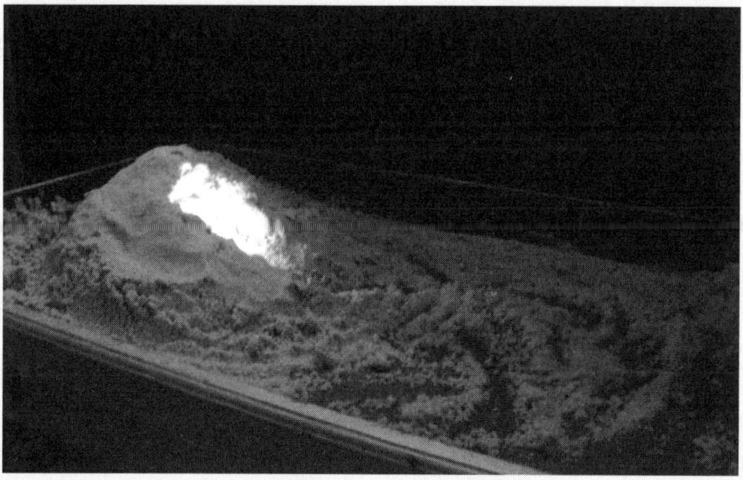

*Figure 1.1 Sandworld*

Down the corridor, behind the door, the room
grows large as it gathers up the dark
ripens into night.
Inside, a flame is beating, breathing, exhaling saplight
on and on into the deepening afternoon.

Molecule by humming molecule, darkness
assembles, knows the day pallid glow
as radiance,
with grave courtesy pays courtly homage,
enters the dance.

## A BRIEF LOOK AT SANDPLAY THERAPY

In 1911 H.G. Wells wrote a small book entitled *Floor Games.* 'The jolliest indoor games for boys and girls demand a floor,' he writes, 'and the home that has no floor upon which games may be played, falls so far short of happiness' (1911/2005, p.38). He describes how, over a span of many years, he and his two sons built whole cities and islands on the green cork carpet of one room of their house, using a vast array of found materials and miniature replicas of buildings and people, animals, railway rails, bricks, boards, and planks. *Floor Games* is a book that reports on delight. For Wells, this play 'not only keep[s] boys and girls happy for days together', but is a rich source for their adult lives, for it 'build[s] up a framework of inspiring ideas in them for after life' (ibid.).

Inspired by Wells' account, the British child psychiatrist Margaret Lowenfeld introduced a cabinet of miniature objects and found materials to her clinic in 1929. The children in her practice began to call the cabinet 'the world'. Lowenfeld then introduced a sandtray. Within two months the children were spontaneously placing into the tray the miniatures that were housed in the cabinet. The children were creating worlds in the sand. The psychiatrist celebrated their activity and provided the conditions in which it would flourish. Her stance is reminiscent of what Froebel, an educator in the previous century, describes to teachers as 'following the child' (1826/2005, p.7). It was children in the clinic who combined sandtray and miniatures, and Lowenfeld who examined, understood, harnessed, and developed their impulse into a therapeutic modality. Lowenfeld called the technique the 'World Technique' (Mitchell and Friedman 1994, p.5).

In years subsequent to its inception, practitioners with different theoretical orientations adapted the technique to a variety of settings. The Swiss therapist Dora Kalff (1980) had a profound impact on its development. Kalff went to London, studied under Lowenfeld, and subsequently added the rich, layered understanding of Carl Jung about symbols, archetypes, and the language of the unconscious. Kalff named the technique sandplay.[3]

3 For a comprehensive outline of the development of sandplay therapy, see Stewart 1990, Thompson 1990, and Mitchell and Friedman 1994.

The effectiveness of sandplay as therapy is contingent on the child's sense of his work as protected both by the confines of sandtray and by the containment of a trusted therapist who creates an environment of safety and acceptance. The sandplay therapist has been trained in awareness of transference and counter-transference factors at work, the symbolic meaning of the miniatures and their placement in the tray, and the trajectory of the process. Kay Bradway (2006) defines three hallmarks of classical sandplay therapy: the creating of a succession of trays, delayed interpretation in which the therapist avoids verbal analysis of the pictures until after completion of the series of trays, and a concurrent process in which talk therapy takes place alongside the sandworld creations.

In the account of their work with children who have experienced trauma, Miller and Boe (1990) demonstrate that children offered sandplay therapy can express their fears, confront the material of their life, and rework traumatic experience at an individual pace, the emotion accompanying the play rendered manageable, because the play itself makes use of symbols that stand in for their feelings and experience. They show that children rework a theme by returning repeatedly to the same storyline and same archetypal figures, slowly changing the story as they revisit it, ultimately enabling a final resolution.

## BACK IN THE CLASSROOM

I recall crossing the border into the United States at Buffalo one morning and being queried by the border guard: this sandplay conference I said that I would be attending – what was it about? I began a careful and long-winded explanation. He looked mystified.

Responding to his perplexity, my husband offered a pithy comment: 'It is a form of psychotherapy.'

'Thank you, sir,' the border guard replied to my husband, his eyes clearing. 'She lost me at "The Unconscious"!'

You, as classroom teacher and special education teacher, may sympathize with the border guard. I am a teacher, not a depth psychologist, you may say. The fact is that sandplay therapy within the classroom is *not* what the school can offer to students. Sandtray play within the classroom is an adaptation of only the first of Bradway's above-mentioned hallmarks of sandplay: the making of a series of sandworlds. Teachers cannot offer interpretation of sand pictures, nor can we offer talk therapy. It is for this reason this book discusses sandtray play within a workshop setting, not sandplay therapy.

But it is evident that a sandtray opportunity within the classroom setting does provide children with a wide territory in which to express and sort out feelings through the activities of symbolic play. At the same time, the play enables students to tap into a fund of creative energy as they discover the stories they carry within.

## Developing social, emotional, and academic skills

It is not the provenance of child psychotherapy alone to build emotional and psychological health; it is a central responsibility in education. And it is not a new challenge. In 1895, in his *Plan of Organization of the University Primary School*, John Dewey writes: 'The ultimate problem of all education is to coordinate the psychological and the social factors' (as cited in Tanner 1997). If schools have a key function in producing students who are characterized by academic, emotional, and social competence, they must look for approaches that encompass the whole child. Limited resources of time and money, as well as the ever more insistent pressure to augment academic performance, increase the need for approaches such as sandtray play that engage both intellect and emotion.

Both psychotherapist and teacher are in the business of providing the conditions whereby children can develop the fullness of their own potential. Both are gardeners, providing the tools and creating an environment in which the native human impulse to growth can flourish. Froebel called his school the 'kindergarten' (garden of children) and writes: 'It is the destiny and life-work of all things to unfold their essence' (1826/2005, p.1). The psychotherapist has the same vision. 'Given the proper conditions,' asserts the sandplay therapist Estelle Weinrib, 'the psyche will heal itself' (1983, p.1).

The summer plant, given the right soil, light, and water, becomes a healthy rose or iris, or elderberry bush. The schoolroom can be a garden in which the riotous design of nature can thrive and each child can express her individuality. By allowing a confluence of the wisdom streams of both education and psychology, we can create conditions whereby children grow up into their own potentiality – where they blossom into the fullness of health, where their innate yearning for connection finds fulfillment.

The fact is that it is futile to try to separate cognitive from emotional and behavioural realities. They are interrelated. The ability to be aware of feelings, control impulses, adapt to circumstances, manage conflict, and sense other people's emotions and react suitably – all these are what Daniel Goleman (1998) described as attributes belonging to emotional intelligence. Teachers and parents presume rightly that social and emotional intelligence leads to academic success. Extensive research corroborates these intuitions (Eisenberg 2006; Guerra and Bradshaw 2008; Masten and Coatsworth 1998; Weissberg and Greenberg 1998 – as cited in Durlak *et al.* 2011).

## The oral language link

But the concomitant reality is that the reverse is also true – academic competence in the area of language fosters social and emotional intelligence. With the capacity both to speak and listen, dialogue becomes possible. Social competence and emotional wellbeing begin to flourish.

Oral language is not confined to the domain of public speaking, a fact of which we are reminded in a staff meeting, a parent/teacher conference, a dinner party, or an estate agent's office. Oral language is the coin of exchange. Those who are flexible users of it are able to navigate nimbly the demands of everyday life.

Many students who get into repeated quarrels are in that pattern of interacting with others because they cannot translate their experience into words. They can neither pinpoint their own feelings, nor receive another's point of view through listening, nor organize their language to describe their own experience. As David Booth observes, 'Just because children arrive at school with some development in this area, we cannot take talk – the integration of listening and speaking – for granted' (2009, p.20). Margaret Donaldson writes that the child 'must become not just able to talk. But to choose what he will say... His conceptual system must expand in the direction of increasing ability to represent itself. He must become capable of manipulating symbols' (as cited in Wells 1986, p.158). Children need to gain mastery over a tool that is used in the service of representing what they want to communicate. They need to learn to command the apparatus of oral language.

Conversation, entreaty, confession, complaint, and persuasion: all belong to the realm of oral language and in each we interact with one another through our narratives. As Robert Fulford (1999) observes, 'Assembling facts or incidents into tales is the only form of expression and entertainment that most of us enjoy equally at age three and age seventy-three' (p.x). Every time we answer the question 'How was your day?' (or 'Your vacation?' or 'Your visit to the dentist?' or 'What happened there?'), we are engaging in the art of creating story out of experience. When, therefore, we bring students to the storytelling segment of the sandtray workshop, we are introducing them to the royal road of communication. Repeated storytelling develops familiarity and confidence with sequencing events and sorting multitudinous details and feelings into a narrative. The skill can then be generalized and applied in other settings.

Take the schoolyard, for example. A difficult narrative that some students are asked to tell and to hear over and over again is the one told in response to the question 'What just happened?' The question is asked and story recounted when there has been a fight on the playground, and it is a difficult story, not only because it is solicited when emotions are running high but also because experience is, as Robert Fulford writes, 'intensely complicated and hard to recount':

> A story has shape, outlines, limits; an experience blurs at the edges and tends to merge imperceptibly with related experience... Stories, in order to become stories, must be simplified stripped of extraneous details and vagrant feeling. (1999, p.4)

Practice in the workshop with telling and hearing the sandtray narratives of peers equips the child to tell and listen to the story of 'what just happened' on the playground. The ability to frame the account gives the child a sense of control and order over the experiential chaos involved in a playground fight. And it disrupts the cycle of frustration and anger by calming the precipitating factors of miscommunication that often lead to fighting in the first place.[4] Similarly, the listener whose untrained impulse may be to defend or attack learns an alternative stance, that of receptivity. Dialogue and resolution become possible. This is social and emotional intelligence at work.

## What is required

What training do teachers need in order to invite sandtray play into their repertoire of classroom tools? The question is wide of the mark. It is not training that is required, but a conscious attitude of receptivity to the child. Like the non-directive therapist who is effective not because of the wisdom imparted, the information provided, or the advice given, but because of the ability to provide a safe, accepting, supportive, listening environment, the facilitator of the sandtray/storymaking workshop is effective because of an ability to provide a climate of safety for the student. What the teacher needs is respect for the unfolding process of the worlds that are built, a disciplined waiting on the student's creativity, and a simple holding of the workshop space in a stance of quiet attentiveness. 'The guide at the side', not the 'sage on the stage'.

Sandworld building and storymaking is playful work and serious play. Like the scientist's laboratory or the artist's studio, the workshop is a world set apart and requires order and safety for its enterprise. Chapter 2 suggests how to create a nurturing setting and set a behavioural structure. Subsequent chapters look at each segment of the workshop – building, telling, listening, and writing. Each chapter approaches its subject both from a theoretical and practical viewpoint; each is illuminated by student work. The final chapter of the book is an account of how the workshop frame has been adapted to a variety of classroom contexts. Teachers share guidelines that created the conditions for the success of their sandtray narrative projects and examine what worked in the various adaptations. I hope that Chapter 7 will act as an invitation to you, the reader, to take what is presented in this book and apply it to your own situation and the particular needs of the children in your care.

---

4 My thanks to Andrea Slocombe for her observations about the impact of classroom storytelling on the capacity of students for coping with altercations on the playground.

Chapter 2

# INFRASTRUCTURE OF NURTURE AND DISCIPLINE

*'The things we say at the door before we come into the workshop have helped me in the yard when I get teased.'*

– Dana, Grade 5 (age ten)

Come inside the workshop. It is January. Light is slanting into the classroom off the frozen ice of the bay. On the windowsills, pink and red geraniums bloom in boxes brought off the deck at the end of summer. Mozart is playing. The time is 11.20 in the morning. One by one, I greet the students who shake my hand at the threshold to the room.

Carter, shuffling, hitches his belt to reign in oversized pants, his booming voice suddenly shy: 'I'll need your help today.'

Gavin offers a simple declaration: 'I am feeling capable today.'

Hugh frowns. His eyes scan the hall and the waiting line: 'I can help others.'

'Mrs. Smith, today I am going to build about the dog's birthday.'

'Good morning, Mrs. Smith. You do not know what King Snake is going to do! Oh no. I won't tell you yet. It will frighten you.'

Lucy may surprise me: 'Today I do not want to build; I know what I want to write. I just want to write my story.'

Darcie, still smarting from politics of the playground, refuses to shake my hand. She crosses her arms, narrows her eyes, and looks away. In five minutes, I hear a knock at the door. Lured by a world waiting to be built, she is ready to give me her message: 'I belong here.'

Inside the workshop, it is the moment of intensity, peace. The wordless humming hangs in the air. It is the sound of children sinking deep into concentration as they deliberate, choose, and design. I take a deep breath. Again, it has happened. The children are in the safety of their own sandtray, supreme in the god-like role of world-makers. The sound in the workshop is not unlike the sound in the centre of a forest. It is a condition of complete activity and complete rest.

## ENTERING AND LEAVING THE WORKSHOP: RITUALS OF GREETING AND FAREWELL

Out of their solitude, builders daydream their worlds. Their play is personal, completely individual, and introverted. In solitude, students encounter and sort out what is within, and discover their stories.[1] For the workshop to be viable, we must help students make the transition from the mode of sociability to the mode of silence. A ritual of greeting marks the transition into the workshop space, orients participants to an inward focus by helping them activate awareness of their own needs and feelings, and imbues the workshop with an atmosphere of acceptance and courtesy. The greeting ritual is mirrored at the end of the session with the farewell ritual. The students put away their portfolios, sweep their space, and close their sandtrays. One by one they shake the teacher's hand, say goodbye, and name what they have learned or accomplished that day in the workshop. The two rituals of greeting and farewell mirror each other: they bookend the workshop with care, respect, and attuned connection. The introductory greeting

1 The importance of safe and secluded space was explored in 1936 by Christiana Morgan in the 'Thematic Apperception Test' (as cited in Douglas 1993). Douglas notes that she 'wrote about the enclosed space as a haven…to which one could retreat from the "dangerous turmoil" of the world and within which creativity could bloom… She traced the fantasy back to a longing to be safely contained within a nurturing mother's arms…"where he or she could daydream, ruminate, and escape from extraverted demands"' (p.205).

sets the tone; the farewell reinforces it. Together they foster a climate of civility within the classroom.

In the exchanges at the door, the teacher is modeling, and the student rehearsing, the act of being courteous to another person. 'Courtesy', I once heard said, 'is simply a way of relating that says to the other, "You are important"'. Situated as we are in a reality television culture where the story of winners and losers frames the creative arts of dancing, cooking, clothing design, and singing, our students are acclimatized to an ethos of judgment. Our classrooms all too often can reinforce that sensibility. By contrast, the rituals of greeting and farewell formulate a climate of acceptance, openness, and interest. They challenge judgment and act as a corrective to it.

## Developing attuned connection

Simone Weil reminds us that, in the Grail legend, the person who asks the wounded king 'What are you going through?' is the one to whom the Grail belongs. When teachers – who both by practice and necessity are skilled multi-taskers – stop, shake hands, and listen to the greeting or farewell of a single student, they are engaged in a Grail-like exchange. Weil describes the attentiveness of the action:

> This way of looking is first of all attentive. The soul empties itself of all its own contents in order to receive into itself the being it is looking at, just as he is, in all his truth. Only he who is capable of attention can do this. (1951, p.115)

Weil is describing the moment when we shelve our own preoccupations in order to make space for another, opening the way to a real connection with him.

Weil's account of the importance of regarding another with attention is being confirmed by contemporary studies in interpersonal neurobiology – the study of how brains affect each other during relationship. Burgeoning research is examining the human being as a social creature, hardwired for relationship. As the psychobiologist Cozolino argues, there is no such thing as a healthy yet isolated brain. The 'living brain [must be] embedded within a community of other brains: relationships are our natural habitat' (2006, p.11).

An individual brain depends upon the brains with which it comes into contact. One effect of this interdependence is what the neuropsychologist Allan Schore describes as the 'interactive regulation of emotion' (2009, p.117). The human capacity to regulate emotions does not happen unilaterally, but in relationship.

A crucial relationship for us is one that the interpersonal neurobiologist Daniel Siegel describes as that of 'attuned connection'. Siegel defines attuned connection as one in which we 'feel felt' by the other. 'Attuned connections,' he writes, are those in which we feel we are 'held within another person's internal world, in their head and in their heart' (2011, p.167). Human beings need these relations with other human beings as we need water and food. The researcher John Bowlby (1988) shows that these connections are crucial in the establishing of secure attachment and a sense of safety in the young child, that being held within the consistent, accepting regard of a parent or primary caregiver gives the child the capacity to be alone and to explore new or uncomfortable situations.

Significantly for teachers, the child who lacked a formative experience of attuned connection, and who therefore has not developed a secure attachment, can develop later what Daniel Siegel calls an 'earned secure attachment'. The 'earned secure attachment' emerges through a positive relationship with a caring adult, giving the child 'a sense of herself as real and valuable even in the face of the chaotic parental environment at home' (2011, p.188). This is good news. Perhaps this is the Holy Grail of teaching.

By being unequivocally available to the child in those brief moments of attentive greeting and farewell, the teacher is engendering a sense of safety in the child. The adult's attentive receptivity supports the child as he enters into the workshop's silence and supports him as he departs. As this pattern of interaction is repeated day after day, the child may develop a sense of security and may build the capacity for self-regulation of emotional reactions. The student's sense of stress may calm, and resourcefulness and curiosity begin to flourish. One student wrote after four months in the sandtray narrative workshop: 'This group is a place where I know I belong and the people here understand the pain I feel sometimes. I feel understood.' His sense of the workshop as a safe and protected space, where he felt connected and understood, had its origins in the structured interactions of the entrance and the exit.

## Exploring the entry ritual

The structured solitude of sandtray play signals a shift in the school day. Hour after hour, relating to others has been the enterprise – playing, competing, loving, fighting, excluding, negotiating – the 'social curriculum' running alongside the academic one. Now, in order to build a sandworld, a child must drop pressing concerns about what others are doing, saying, and thinking, must withdraw from the fray, must leave behind the voices of *He butted me... Will you play with me next break?... Why can't I be the goalie?... I want to be on your team... Will you be my friend?... It's my turn to be first.* Silence can feel uncomfortably foreign for our children whose lives are lived in the noise of television, the chatter of texting, the relentless programming of before-and-after-school extracurricular activities. The entrance ritual provides support to students making a transition to quiet.

The students wait outside the workshop. One by one, the teacher invites them to the threshold of the classroom to shake hands, grounding the interaction in a physical exchange. A menu of possible messages is affixed to the doorway (Figure 2.1). The student chooses one message from the menu, or a pressing thought, feeling, or expectation, and shares it with the teacher. The threshold to the workshop is a demarcation line. Each enters the workshop in solitude.

By comparison to our culture's ritualized greeting and response of 'How are you?' and 'Fine thank you', the exchange at the workshop door gives the child a moment when she comes home to herself, an opportunity to touch base with feelings and needs. *What message will be true about me today?* The child must decide the answer to that question, hear her own voice speaking her needs, feelings, or goals. The authority of the others must give way to the authority of her singular person. What has transpired previously is left outside. The child enters into dedicated space, one set apart for work and expression.

### *The content of the entry messages*

'The things we say at the door before we come in to the workshop have helped me in the yard when I get teased,' 11-year-old Dana reflects, a few months into the sandtray play. The content of the messages has stayed with her and sustained her beyond the doors of the classroom. I believe that one reason for this is that the menu of messages (seen in Figure 2.1) from which the child chooses a threshold greeting is a resource that meets developmental needs.

THE MESSAGE MENU OF THE ENTRY

I am feeling capable today.
I will need your help today.
I belong here.
I can think clearly.
I can learn the rules that help me live with others.
I can learn many new things.
I can help others.
I can be responsible for my behaviour.
I am feeling many feelings.
I can explore and experiment and be interested in everything.

*Figure 2.1 Menu of greeting messages provided to students upon entering the workshop*

Erikson (1963, 1968) asserts that humans go through predictable stages of development. He calls them the 'eight ages of man' (1963, p.247). Like a house, a personality is constructed floor by floor. Each stage has its own challenge or 'crisis', in the sense of 'turning point', in the 'ever new configuration that is the growing personality' (1968, p.96). Erikson argues that the successful resolution of the crisis of each stage means that the child is able to go forth into the succeeding stage with the 'strength' or 'virtue' gained by that resolution (1968, p.234).

The foundational level, according to Erikson, is *Hope*, a strength that is forged through the successful resolution of the initial life challenge of *Trust vs. Mistrust* faced by the infant. *Initiative* and *Guilt* need to be experienced by the kindergarten child for the strength of *Purpose* to emerge. The six- to twelve-year-old students of our elementary schools are working through the developmental crisis of *Industry vs. Inferiority* as they deal with tasks related to academic performance and peer social interaction. A successful negotiation of that stage, according to Erikson, leads to *Competence.* Hope, self-control, willpower, direction, purpose, competence (1963, p.274) – this is a list of some strengths or virtues that Erikson posits are achieved by the successful resolution of each stage. The list presages the traits we are seeking to foster in our current character education initiatives.[2]

It is clear that we cannot drill moral and performance character traits into children through intellect alone. The traits are not a set of clothes to be put on, but are woven into the warp and woof of the person. They are not memorized and performed; rather they are earned in the emotional and visceral struggles of life. It is imperative, then, that we do not merely lecture our children, but support them in the work of their developmental crises. To do this work of support, we can articulate messages that encourage children in meeting the challenges of each stage. The messages that we give children influence how they negotiate and make meaning of their experience.

The parent educators Jean Illsley Clarke and Connie Dawson (1998) contend that if the adults in a child's life understand that one stage is not the same as another, they can give the child informed and appropriate support. The 16-month-old who explores all the nooks and crannies of the house, the five-year-old who wears his Superman cape all day, and the 11-year-old who is disagreeing with us are each doing the work of their stage. This is inconvenient for the adult perhaps, but our task is to understand their fledgling attempts for what they are and to help children to practise and refine the skills they are developing.

Messages that give children permission to undertake stage-specific work will help equip them to do tasks required by those stages. In answer to the child's unspoken questions of 'Who am I in relation to others?' and 'How do I acquire the skills that I need?' (1998, p.212), Clarke and Dawson designed a series of affirmations specifically tailored to support and encourage the child in the developmental work of the stages, which they name Being, Doing, Thinking, Identity, and Structure. The messages they designed for the developing child are seen in Figure 2.2.

2 See, for example, Character Education Partnership (2008) *Performance Values: Why They Matter and What Schools Can Do to Foster Their Development.*

**Being:** *birth to six months* *Developmental task:* **Deciding to live**
*I am glad you are alive; You belong here; What you need is important to me; I'm glad you are you; You can grow at your own pace; You can feel all of your feelings; I love you and I care for you willingly.*

---

**Doing:** *six to 18 months* *Developmental task:* **Starting to do things on our own**
*You can explore and experiment and I will support and protect you; You can use all of your senses when you explore; You can do things as many times as you need to; You can know what you know; You can be interested in everything; I like to watch you initiate and grow and learn; I love you when you are active and when you are quiet.*

---

**Thinking:** *18 months to three years* *Developmental task:* **Deciding it's okay to think**
*I am glad you are starting to think for yourself; It's okay for you to be angry and I won't let you hurt yourself or others; You can say no and push and test limits as much as you need to; You can learn to think for yourself and I will learn to think for myself; You can think and feel at the same time; You can know what you need and ask for help; You can become separate from me and I will continue to love you.*

---

**Identity:** *three to six years* *Developmental task:* **Learning who we are**
*You can explore who you are and find out who other people are; You can be powerful and ask for help at the same time; You can try out different roles and ways of being powerful; You can find out the results of your behaviour; All of your feelings are okay with me; You can learn what is pretend and what is real; I love who you are.*

---

**Structure:** *six to 12 years* *Developmental task:* **Learning to do things our own way**
*You can think before you say yes or no and learn from your mistakes; You can trust your intuition to help you decide what to do; You can find a way of doing things that works for you; You can learn the rules that help you live with others; You can learn when and how to disagree; You can think for yourself and get help instead of staying in distress; I love you even when we differ; I love growing with you.*

*From* Growing Up Again *(Second Edition) by Jean Illsley Clarke, Connie Dawson. Copyright 1989, 1998 by Hazelden Foundation. Reprinted by permission of Hazelden Foundation, Center City, MN.*

*Figure 2.2 Developmental ages, stages, tasks, and affirmations*

The messages of the entrance menu (Figure 2.1) are excerpted from the whole spectrum of Clarke and Dawson's catalog in the *Growing Up Again* (1998) series. The messages are provided not only for the needs of six- to twelve-year-olds, but address the needs of every developmental stage. There are two reasons for this:

- Not every child resolves the challenges of developmental stages within the allotted time frame. Sometimes a stage is not successfully negotiated the first time around. Many of our six- to twelve-year-olds need to return to tasks of previous stages in order to finish developmental work (Clark and Dawson 1998; Levin 1988). Although our students may be in the six- to twelve-year-old range, they may need to affirm messages geared to earlier stages if they are recycling the challenges of those stages.
- Sometimes a new challenge reopens a need to hear an old affirmation. A difficulty in the present moment may echo the challenge of an earlier stage. For example, 'Can the world be trusted?' may be a question that a child asks again when a new life situation threatens equilibrium or sense of security. He may need to hear again the affirmations for the foundational stage of birth to six months.

In speaking their chosen message out loud to a comprehending ear, children will hear the words they need to hear and feed their hunger for an affirmation that will help them negotiate or recycle developmental tasks. The content of the messages meets deep needs. One of my students, who recently had been adopted as a five-year-old out of an environment of early neglect, chose unfailingly, day after day, week after week, the message addressed to those negotiating the initial stage of *Being*: 'I belong here.' His tentative first attempts at writing emerged as he copied the affirmation; then recopied it with the names of each family member. Finally, in a generosity born of his desire to feel the words – the thrill of them and the truth they point to – he made a book. Beside the photograph of each classmate, on each page, the affirmation was repeated over and over: *Jimmy belongs here. Rahim belongs here. Gabriella belongs here...* This was his mantra, his story, his heartbeat.

## Exploring the ritual of farewell

As students shake hands and say goodbye at the end of the workshop, they articulate what they are thinking or feeling about what they accomplished or learned that day. They provide a snapshot of their thoughts, a one-sentence summary of what stood out for them:

- A new learning: *I was able to get to the point when I tell my story.*
- A satisfaction: *My favourite part was telling my story.*
- An observation about personal process or style of working: *I really think that it is easier to write my story than to tell it. When I tell it, I get confused.*
- An observation about behaviour: *Tomorrow I will try to stay in my own space the whole time I am building.*
- An intention for the next workshop: *I want to stay with the same world next time. Tomorrow I want to make the king arrive.*
- Some messages indicate the student is still ruminating about the shared reading: *I think I know what Sylvester is going to do to get unfrozen.*[3]

Satisfaction, expectation, reflection, realization, intention: the students leave these behind at their departure, to be retrieved when they return and used as signposts that orient them to the work of the next session.

### *Metacognition*

Metacognition is the word we give to what the students practise in the farewell ritual. *Meta* is from the Greek, meaning 'greater than' or 'beyond'. The students are doing 'greater than' thinking when they step outside the recent experience, reflect on it, and make plans from it. They are thinking about their thinking. The Ontario government's document *Growing Success* calls this assessment *as* learning. 'Assessment *as* learning,' it states, 'is information that is used by students to... monitor their own progress towards achieving their own learning

3 Referring to the shared reading mentor text of *Sylvester and the Magic Pebble* (Steig 1969).

goals...make adjustments in their learning approaches, reflect on their learning, and set individual goals for learning' (Ontario Ministry of Education 2010, p.31).

The students leave with a spoken realization of what they have accomplished. That one-sentence summary of their experience acts as a brief, preparing them for the next workshop. It gives rise to strategic thinking, a type of thinking that can become part of their repertoire when approaching any area of the curriculum.

The skills of metacognitive thinking do not emerge automatically. Over the span of the initial weeks of the workshop, the teacher models repeatedly the sound of this kind of thinking in comments such as 'You did a great job today on adding detail to your telling. Tomorrow you are going to be ready to unpack your ending' or 'I saw that you were very focused during the building today. I am just waiting to see what you do next in your world.' This modeling not only reinforces the student's awareness of the teacher's regard, but also demonstrates evaluation and specific goal setting in action. Gradually over time, the teacher releases to the student the responsibility for the farewell message.

## INSIDE THE WORKSHOP: GUIDELINES FOR SOLITUDE AND INTERACTION

The workshop proper, like its entrance and exit, requires a conscious frame of caring and structure. Sandtray play and storymaking is a two-phase enterprise – the solitude and quiet of the building phase followed by the interaction of story sharing and responding. Workshop guidelines for the participants address the requirements for solitude as well as for sharing, providing the needed discipline and nurture for both phases.

### Guidelines for solitude

There are two rules for the building phase of the workshop. Both rules create the conditions for individual work in solitude. Both rules are couched in a positive voice. Instead of 'Don't intrude', the rule is

'You are in your own workspace'. Instead of 'No talking', the rule is 'The only sound we hear is Mozart'.

## Maintaining the space

*You are in your own workspace!* When entering a sandtray workshop, the students enter a psychological bubble in which they can play out their own stories, hear their own voice, create their own worlds. The first rule promotes awareness that the individual workspace has boundaries. This rule is particularly important when the physical constraints of the classroom mean that students are building in close proximity to one another, a situation that occurs inevitably when the workshop is offered to an entire class of students in one room simultaneously. 'You are in your own workspace' becomes the imperative that orients students psychologically to the need for solitude, cueing them to give sole attention to their own sandtrays and individual bags of miniatures (Figure 2.3).

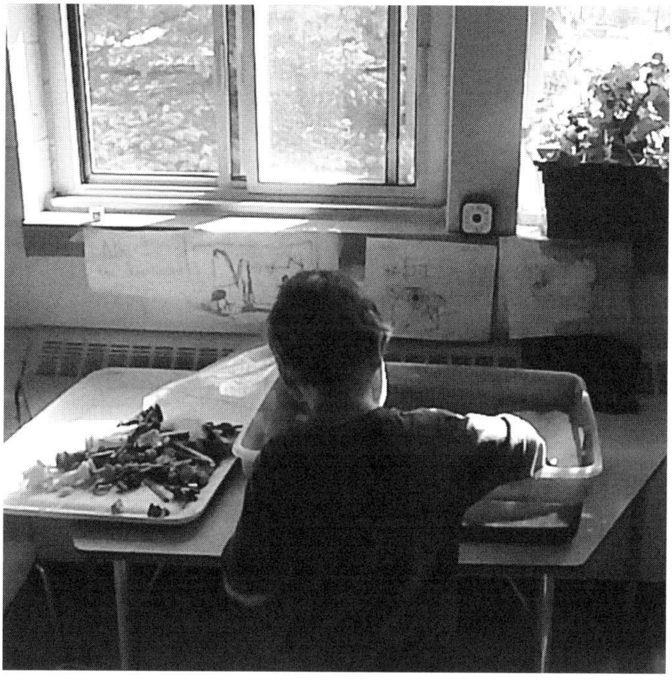

*Figure 2.3 'You are in your own workspace'*

### *Honouring the quiet*

*The only sound we hear is Mozart!* In her book *The Soul of Education,* Rachael Kessler (2000) points out that silence does not necessarily bring children immediate equilibrium; instead, silence may invite inner emotional turmoil to the surface, where children can deal with it consciously, sift through it, name it, sort it out, and identify it. Identifying feelings, Kessler also reminds us, is 'a basic capacity in emotional intelligence – the foundation of all other emotional and social skills' (p.39). Uncomfortable for some students, the silence of the building phase provides the environment in which emotional intelligence may be fostered. In the workshop, the harmony and order of classical music plays as a backdrop to the silence of the world making, companioning the children in their journey into places that may contain turmoil.

The regulation of play by music is a notion as old as Plato: 'the love for law enters [children's] souls with the music accompanying the games, never leaves them and helps in their development' (cited by W.N. Hailmann in Froebel 2005, p.57). By virtue of its measured cadences and mathematical progressions, classical music offers an organized sound that both energizes and calms. Madeleine L'Engle (1980) writes: 'Surely [children's] passion for the Pachelbel canon is a passion for order in a disordered world. And they love the combination of order and delight in a Bach fugue' (p.140).

Barth writes that Mozart:

> heard the harmony of creation to which the shadow also belongs but in which the shadow is not darkness... Mozart has created order for those who have ears to hear, and he has done it better than any scientific deduction could (1978, p.69).

There is a body of research that reveals that listening to music enhances the density of neural circuits in the primary auditory cortex, and that grey matter – the part of the brain responsible for information processing – tends to be more concentrated in musicians (cited in Levitin 2006). At the very least, playing classical music contributes to the felt sense of the workshop as time set apart. It introduces an abstract and soothing quality; it enfolds the space with clarity and peacefulness.

## Guidelines for interaction

The silence of the building segment is followed by interactive phases of the workshop: telling, listening, and responding to the sandtray story. Rules for the interactive phase address the matters of relating to peers and working within the workshop and are posted for ready reference on the workshop wall.

### *Relating to others*

*'No hurts!' 'Stick together!'* Borrowed from the work of Phyllis Rubin outlined in 'Group Theraplay' (2001, p.367), the rules of 'No hurts!' and 'Stick together!' define the attitude required from the participants during group mini-lessons and peer conferencing. The two rules are one and the same rule. 'Stick together' reframes in the positive voice what the first rule, 'No hurts', states in the negative. Together, the two injunctions comprise one guideline for relating that forms a touchstone for the atmosphere of courtesy, respect, and supportiveness upon which the workshop relies.

### *Approaching the task*

*'Work hard!'* is the second injunction. It addresses the seriousness of the expectation that we have for the students. Sandtray play is work, and when the story is told, the communicating of it in words also is work. 'Work hard' identifies and dignifies this reality for the participants.

## WHEN ADDITIONAL STRUCTURE IS REQUIRED

Sometimes the guidelines outlined above need to be supplemented. A group of students who are particularly frenetic may require further supports to ensure an orderly entry. An individual student who is severely disruptive or displays oppositional behaviour may require additional individual structures designed to meet her needs.

## When a group needs additional preparation upon entry

- Needing support to calm down prior to the greeting ritual, the students in a particularly unruly group of primary-age children should be assigned a personal place in the entrance line of the hallway. Designating boundaries is a way of containing the behaviour for those who are in a habit of intruding on others' personal space.
- In the hallway prior to the workshop entrance, lead the group in Brain Gym®, a centring and calming strategy. A technique developed by Paul and Gail Dennison (1986), Brain Gym® helps to integrate both sides of the brain through physical exercises and movement repatterning.
- The sequence finishes with a visualization exercise in which students close their eyes and cross their arms and ankles. It is helpful to take the students through a visualization that might sound like the following:
    - Make a picture in your head.
    - Picture yourself in your own office with your own sandtray. The only sound you are hearing is the sound of Mozart and the sound of the sand.
    - Picture yourself building a world, telling the story of that world to your partner, and listening to your partner's story.
    - How are you feeling? What is your plan? Decide on the message you want to give to me today when you enter the workshop.

  - When you have a picture in your head and you know how you are feeling and your plan for today, unhook your arms and legs and I will invite you into the classroom.[4]

## When individual students need additional structure

Hugo would come into class with good intentions, but perfectionism and frustration at the gap between his telling and its record fueled verbal outbursts, ripping up of stories, and, on one despairing day, the tearing apart of his entire portfolio. We tried to address the frustration in various ways – scribing for him as he told the story, modifying the writing requirement, and encouraging the use of assistive technology – but the bottom line was that Hugo needed to learn to participate in the civility of the workshop. He was negotiating what Erikson characterized as the developmental crisis of *Industry vs. Inferiority* (1968, p.94). How could we help him achieve a sense of competence? We knew that he needed to develop internal structure. He needed to internalize the rule of 'Work hard'.

'School is your work,' we insisted, 'and as such you need to finish it, just the same as your father must complete his work at his office. Time wasted during work has to be made up.'

Paying back time for time that has been wasted appeals to a sense of justice. It is logical and fair. 'School is your job' gives gravitas to children's effort. One day in early March, we logged the time Hugo spent off task and arranged for him to pay it back in his own time. When he entered the resource classroom that afternoon, I handed Hugo a rubric and asked him to set behaviour goals for the time he was to spend there that day. They could be anywhere from a Level 1 to a Level 4. They encompassed such categories as independent work, initiative, and responsibility. Hugo was to mark descriptors that best articulated his goals for that day and, in so doing, set out to achieve

4 Some workshops use the Brain Gym® sequence not at the outset as a prelude to the greeting but as an effective movement and refocusing break in mid-workshop, as a demarcation between building and sharing, or as an introductory activity in the mini-lesson. As students become practised with the routine, they are able to direct their peers through the movement sequence, rotating the coveted position of leadership.

them. At the end of his minutes of repayment, I would sign the rubric in the descriptor that best reflected what his actual behaviour had been. It would go home for sharing with his parents.

That first afternoon, Hugo was hooked. He looked at the possible behaviours he might choose and set his goal at a lofty Level 4. Sure enough, he jumped into his work with both feet. At the end of the 33-minute time debt repayment, he took home a rubric on which I had corroborated his accomplishment. The following morning Hugo brought the paper back with a signature and message of celebration from his parent. In the hallway he shook my hand and said, 'And I want one every day.'

Day by day the rubric was anchor and motivator. At the outset of the sandtray workshop, Hugo stamped the category that best articulated his behaviour goals; at random intervals during the class, both he and I checked where we observed his actual behaviours to be, and at the end of class I initialed the category that reflected his overall effort. His parent in turn signed the paper and sent it back to school, often with a message of encouragement, sometimes with disappointment. The data began to accumulate in his writer's portfolio; he was building up evidence of a good work ethic. No words, no verbal reminders were required to bring him back to the task at hand: the piece of paper was a reminder of his own best vision and pointing to it brought him back to it.

It turned out that when Nell saw this in action, she decided that was what she wanted also. She had struggled with buying into the rule 'Work hard' for her own reasons. She had found that the attention she craved could be elicited by spilling sand, intruding on others during writing time, and spreading the boundaries of her workspace physically into others' space. When she requested a behaviour rubric for herself, she was demonstrating that she knew better than we did what she really craved – positive attention. From that time it formed the base from which Nell engaged in the workshop. The combination of experiencing a logical consequence for breaking the rule (paying back time), together with the opportunity to predetermine the level of achievement in following it, built the capacity to accept structure. She began to explore what it felt like to be adequate to the task.

What was it that motivated Hugo and Nell to connect to the rubric and be prepared to adopt it? We cannot know but we can take some guesses:

- The requirement for nightly parent signature meant that the child was accountable at home and school. School and home were working together. The child's world made sense.
- 'Mistaken goals of their misbehaviour' (Dreikurs 1964, p.58) were met in a positive way. Hugo was caught off-guard. The mode of confrontation, comfortably familiar to him, was depotentiated because we were saying to him that, insofar as he could determine how he met the non-negotiable rule of 'Work hard', he could be the boss. For Nell, attention from the teacher during random check-ins during the workshop, and from parents when they read and responded to the rubric, seemed to inspire her subsequent efforts and successes.
- The rubric was a form of encouragement because it assumed achievement. It opened the door to a world in which success was expected.
- The rubric defined 'Work hard'. With its descriptors, it taught that achievement was the process not product. The process was within reach. All a student had to do was to show up and try.
- The rubric said tacitly that a level of complete excellence might not be possible or even desirable every single day. It gave Hugo and Nell permission to acknowledge that their capacity varied.
- The rule 'Work hard' was non-negotiable. Both students learned to see it as relevant, to internalize it, and, in so doing, change an attitude of 'I can't do it' to 'I can learn from my mistakes'. It may seem that it moved the locus of control away from the teacher, but in reality control was shared: the student's freedom was exercised within parameters defined by the teacher.

Chapter 3

# BUILDING

*'Mother Nature would be my hands.'*

– Marina, Grade 4 (age nine)

*'I don't know how the story goes if I don't do it with my hands. My body does the story.'*

– Abel, Grade 4 (age nine)

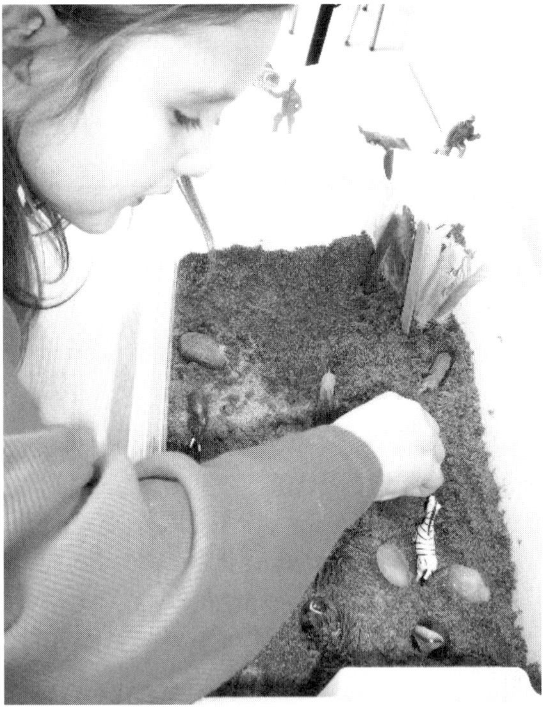

*Figure 3.1 Building a world*

# WHAT HAPPENS DURING BUILDING?

The student enters the room within a blanket of solitude that the quiet threshold has wrapped around him. He finds at his desk a large bag of miniatures and an empty sandtray. He molds the sand and places miniatures in it that appeal or are meaningful to him. 'He forms hills, tunnels, plains, lakes, and rivers in the sand, just as he views the world from his own situation, and he allows the figures to act as he experiences them in his fantasy,' writes Kalff (1980, p.39). He creates something new. What is going on during this act of creation, we wonder.

## Expressing without words

'Mother Nature would be my hands,' Marina explains to me. She is pouring water on her world from a recycled yogurt container. A rainstorm is deluging the mountains and lowlands of the sandtray. Now the characters in her world have a new topography to contend with. Peaks are leveled and valleys are flooding – like her life of late, which has been so changed that its former lineaments have been rendered unrecognizable.

'Often the hands will know how to solve a riddle with which the intellect has wrestled in vain,' Jung writes (1969, p.86). 'By shaping it,' he continues, 'the initially incomprehensible, isolated event is integrated into the sphere of total personality.' In the stroke of deluging her world, Marina shapes a model of her feelings. Busy with her hands, immersed in sand and water, she expresses her perplexity. The sandtray might be called a 'mirror world', which, like the 'sacramental' one described by Zimmer (1971), 'catches all the rays sent up from the unconscious and presents them as an external reality susceptible to manipulation' (p.19). Zimmer adds, 'Any considered change of scenery in the tangible...mirror sphere brings about almost automatically, a corresponding shift in the interior field and point of view' (ibid.). The washing out of the world and manipulating the scene of the devastation is for Marina inexplicably satisfying. And, if Zimmer is correct, it may shift her point of view.

## Thinking by means of doing

'I don't know how the story goes if I don't do it with my hands,' Abel tells me. 'My body does the story.' Engrossed, Abel builds, and, by building, he knows his ideas. In Abel's experience, thought and idea come not through writing or talking but through image and movement. This is learning by doing, thinking by acting. This is the play instinct at work more than the intellect at play.

Neumann describes the child at play as his 'total embeddedness in the magical-mythical symbol-world of fantasy and play' (1988, p.70). Abel inhabits his story. From inside his world he is each of the characters. He is judge and judged, king and beggar, brother and sister, superman and little boy, mother and witch, soldier and priest, father and son, hunter and hunted. The story emerges out of the events that these characters initiate and the circumstances to which they respond, the perspectives they bring, their actions, and reactions to each other. Abel is 'embedded' in his sandworld.

## Observing even while participating

Even as he is a participant within his sandworld, Abel stands outside and above it, as the shaper of the scene and orchestrator of the drama. He is observer, overseer, playwright, and director. Kestly points out that this duality is what is singular about sandtray play – the child who is embedded in the play is at the same time able to stand above the play. She writes that 'The miniature sand tray allows the child to be *in* the play and *apart* from the play at the same time'. She calls this doubling the 'participant-observer phenomenon' (2010, p.265).

Students experience a variety of perspectives while in the midst of the play. Observer/director and participant/actors have very different points of view. The challenge of how to tell the story in light of these several standpoints is what the students face as they put their stories into words.

# BUILDING: WHO NEEDS IT?

Strategies typically at work in our classrooms for developing thought and sharing ideas are the strategies of oral and written language, taught with tools such as the ubiquitous blackline master web, chart, and topic list; the oral and written brainstorming activity; and the face-to-face partner sharing. As educators, we must contend with the fact that when these are the only catalysts to generating and sharing ideas, a significant number of our learners opt out. These populations may include children who, because of receptive or expressive language impairment, find the oral language of discussion unrewarding or difficult, and group brainstorming fraught with a sense of isolation and frustration. Others have sensory-motor integration disorders, or difficulties with visual-motor integration, sequential memory, with crossing mid-line, or with hand–eye coordination, with visual-spatial organization, or with processing speed. For these students, the challenge of physically recording their thoughts is formidable and the content of their thinking can be obscured by the effort to write. These children too often begin to believe that they have little to contribute to the classroom, that school itself is a place to which they are not suited.

Sandtray play offers the opportunity to generate ideas without the medium of language. Children discover ideas in the sand, when they engage actively and kinaesthetically with real objects, using what Jerome Bruner (1966) called 'enactive' (action-based) and 'iconic' (image-based) modes of thinking. It is afterwards, as they translate the story into words, that they move on to what Bruner labeled 'symbolic' (language-based) thinking (1996, pp.10–11). Kinaesthetic learners who are given the opportunity to build in order to think, and language-disabled students who can show visually their thinking in order to communicate, begin to regard themselves as contributing members of the classroom community, as having something to say, as possessing of ideas and imagination. Building in the sand addresses a foundational sensory need. For a student who has sensory integration difficulties, the play is grounding; for the kinaesthetic learner, it is a return to native territory because to express through movement is her innate impulse.

Learning from Abel, we can make the suggestion to a child who is at a loss for ideas: 'I don't know what ideas are in you either. So go to the sand and let your body tell you what your ideas are.' Tacitly communicated in our instruction to 'find ideas in the sand' is the message that the student does have them. Our assumption and expectation is that the student is competent, creative, and resourceful. For those who are unable to access ideas through writing or through oral discussion, this expectation comes as a revelation and as revolutionary to their self-concept.

## Sandtray play and boys' literacy learning

One population particularly at risk for school disenchantment is that of young boys. An article in *Maclean's* magazine referencing a recent large-scale National Institutes of Health study of brain development shows that a three-and-a-half-year-old girl's brain is roughly equivalent to that of a five-year-old boy (Intini 2010, p.2). This developmental fact gives girls an advantage in the areas of self-regulation and focus as they start school. 'The net result,' the article says, quoting Leonard Sax, author of *Boys Adrift*, 'is that many boys form a negative conclusion about school early on... And research shows that these attitudes that kids form very early, are very stable... They're set, like concrete.' If boys have the additional burden of sensory-motor or visual-motor difficulties, or language impairment, they are even more seriously at risk for negative attitude towards school. The antidote, according to Sax, is to find a way that makes an 'alternative culture in which it's cool to be smart' (ibid.).

In one school, a group of eight boys whose teachers identified them with observations that included comments about resisting help, having meltdowns, refusing to be scribed for, disengagement in the program, and refusing to participate in class or complete assignments, were chosen to participate in a sandtray narrative program. At the outset of the program the boys articulated their feelings and observations about school and rated various components of their school day on a scale of 1–10. A compilation of the boys' observations is related below. Their frustration and discouragement is palpable in the lines of these interviews. The adjective 'disenchanted' would have been applicable to them.

- About the literacy block:
    - *I'd rather DO stuff than read and write.*
    - *Reading and writing? NEGATIVE 10! I really don't like it.*
    - If *I have an idea it's a 4.*
- About paying attention:
    - *I find it hard to listen for a long time.*
    - *I forget the rules and think about other things.*
    - *I pay attention to things that stay still, but I pay attention better in French because he walks around and uses his hands.*
    - *How much I pay attention depends on the topic math: 10. Writing: 1.*
- About school enjoyment:
    - *School is a 5 because we get gym and art.*
    - *I have fun at recess and gym but I hate reading and writing.*
    - *School is good because I see my buds. But I don't like the work.*
    - *I like gym, math, and science.*

After the boys participated in a sandtray narrative workshop series, they were interviewed again. In their interviews, they revealed a sea change that had taken place in all areas of their school experience. This was not a surprise to the teachers. What was a surprise was the revelation that, over the course of the year, the boys had been continuing their sandtray worlds out into the schoolyard, where in wide games at recess they played out the ideas born in their classroom trays. '*Then,*' they added, '*what we played at recess would influence our stories in class.*' Recess and literacy learning had become reciprocal activities. The playground had become an extension of the classroom.

An alternative culture had been formed in which, in Sax's words, learning was 'cool'.

We might wonder what the students had to say about their experience of sandtray world building. Did they classify it as play or work? What would they tell their peers about the experience of building in the sandtray? Where did the students find the ideas for their worlds? This is how they answered these questions as they looked back on a sandtray play experience.

- Is it play or work?
  - *It is both play and work because you get to play in the sand but you are creating a story at the same time.*
  - *It is playing* while *working which is awesome.*
- How would you describe sandtray play to a classmate?
  - *Building is so fun and awesome because you get to play in the sand but you are still working while you are doing it.*
  - *You are playing, not working, and don't get into trouble.*
  - *It seems easier because you have your hands on it.*
- Where do you get ideas for worlds?
  - *We would get to the sand and just start building and using our hands. The story would come.*
  - *Sometimes we would draw our ideas from what we dream at night.*

## SANDTRAY PLAY: ESSENTIALS FOR BUILDING

Room configuration and the provision of materials form prerequisite physical preparations for the workshop. Timing and a cleanup protocol facilitate the flow of the workshop. The teacher provides a physical and emotional context that invites student expression, and designs record-keeping strategies that enhance and illuminate the building process.

## Room configuration

In the classroom, trays and miniatures must be accessible to a number of sandworld builders simultaneously. The school setting for sandtray play stands in contrast to the sandplay therapy space, which is set up for work with a single client, and where the walls are lined with miniatures, and two wooden sandtrays, one filled with wet sand and the other with dry sand, await one person (Kalff 1980, p.31). In the classroom, the presentation of materials needs to be arranged so their use is practicable for many individuals building in close proximity to each other, within a group setting. Following Janet Escobedo's suggestion (2006), we contain multiple assortments of miniatures within bags and provide multiple sand-filled, stackable plastic trays. By means of individual collections and trays, each student desk becomes a version of the sandtray playroom.

As far as possible, it is necessary to set up the desks to be islands. Cardboard voting booths salvaged from an election or study carrels create visual barriers.

- In settings where it is possible, strategically position the desks in order to foster the sense of interiority. Individualize the space with the name of the child and – as the months progress – photos of the child at work writing, sharing, and building, as well as sandworld maps and story outlines. Display reference sheets of commonly used words and the child's own private stock of important words for quick reference – key words that play a recurring role in their stories: Carter, for example, had 'soldier'; Gavin had 'race car'; Darcie had 'princess' and 'apology'; Gerri had 'whale'.

## Materials

Trays, sand, water, and miniatures are indispensable to the activity of sandworld building. These resources need to be made available individually for each participant. The following sections offer suggestions for acquiring, storing, and distributing the materials of the building phase.

- Sandtrays:
  - Purchase plastic storage containers with fitting lids of 27-litre or 28-quart size, approximately 58.4 cm long by 15.2 cm wide by 15.2 cm high (23 x 16 ¼ x 6 inches).
  - Provide one large plastic container to each student.
  - The trays' lids enable the trays to be stacked in one corner of the classroom or in a storage area when not in use.
  - Spraypaint the inside surface of the containers blue so that the interior of the tray can represent water and sky.
- Sand:
  - Fill the tray to about one-third capacity with sand.
  - Play sand can be purchased from teacher catalogues and from local building supply stores.
  - Sand can vary in texture, colour, and quality, from white sand (which some of my students call 'sugar sand') to coarse sand (which some children have dubbed 'black sand'). Sand texture seems to resonate with various psychological spaces and kind of worlds students want to build on a given day. Typically available play sand is the most practical.
  - In order to prevent mold growth, sand that has been dampened needs to dry before the lid is replaced onto the box.
- Water:
  - Wet sand creates opportunity for tunneling and molding that dry sand does not. It provides a tactile, sensory experience that dry sand does not.
  - An individual student's impulse to flood his world may be therapeutic but it can be disruptive to a large group and problematic for cleanup. Monitor the students' use of water

within the group setting by making water available to the students upon request.

- Storage of miniatures: bags or shoeboxes:
  - Provide one shoebox or large plastic locking bag (38 cm or 15 inches square) to each student.
  - Distribute bags or boxes at random on each student's desk unless a student has specifically requested the same collection as she used in the previous session.
- Miniatures:
  - Most miniatures can be found at the dollar store. Garage sales and Goodwill (charity) stores are worth frequenting for what turns up. Chess pieces serve well as representatives of archetypal and medieval figures.
  - Include in each bag a selection of miniatures from every category listed below. The collections contain miniatures from set categories but each is unique because each contains one-of-a-kind items. The outcome is parallel but distinct collections in individual bags.
  - As the seasons change, add new vegetation and figures and monitor for cleanliness and variety.
  - Do not permit students to exchange figures with each other, as that interrupts the requisite silence.

Categories and examples of miniatures to include in the collections include the following (see Weinrib 1983, p.11):

  - *People:* adults, children, different occupations (sports figures, soldiers, medical, miners, farmers), villains, heroes.
  - *Buildings:* houses, schools, churches, castles.
  - *Animals:* domesticated, wild, zoo, prehistoric, fish, birds, reptiles, mammals.

  - *Fantasy and mythological figures:* mermaids, magicians, movie characters such as Harry Potter or Jaws, cartoon characters such as Garfield, fairy story characters such as Cinderella.
  - *Vehicles:* various modes of transportation – land, air, water, space, war.
  - *Natural objects:* shells, driftwood, stones, sticks, bones, eggs, rocks, feathers, vegetation.
  - *Building materials:* popsicle (lolly) sticks, small blocks, generic shapes, beads. These can be used to create vehicles and structures such as fences, gates, doorways, pathways, bridges, dwellings, and furniture.
  - *Miscellaneous objects:* treasure chests, jewelry, implements, bells.

## Time frame

- Despite diversity in the total available time for a workshop, the building segment requires, at a minimum, 20 minutes.
- Facilitate the builder's transition to the phase of telling the story with a 'five-minute warning'. There need be no large class announcement terminating the building section, but a gentle and individual reminder to wrap up in five minutes.
- Provide a visual cue with a *Time Timer* or draw a clock that shows the end time so that the students see the parameters in which they have to work.

## Cleanup

In the sandplay therapy environment, where it is considered to be crucial to the process that the client leave the playroom with the memory of an intact world, the therapist photographs the sandworld and dismantles it only after the client has left (Weinrib 1983, p.14). In the school setting, constraints of time and space dictate otherwise.

Prior to moving on to the next period, students dismantle their own worlds, brush off the miniatures and replace them in the bags, level the sand, put the lid back on the tray, and sweep up any sand around their desks. When done with a sense of deliberation and care, clearing the tray and smoothing the sand will act as a bridging activity in the setting where participants must transition to the extraverted round of the school day within seconds of leaving the sandplay room. For some students, the dismantling of their world safeguards the sense of privacy and their control over it.

- Sandworlds remain intact during the telling, listening, and writing segments of the workshop. Students dismantle and put away the materials as the culminating activity.
- Allot adequate time for these tasks that bring closure to the session. Students need to dismantle their trays with respect for the worlds that they created and for the miniatures they have used.
- Provide tools for cleanup: dustpan and brush sets, water, and strainers for drying objects that have been rinsed.
- Assign a rotating class monitor or lead cleaner to sweep the entire area and check the desks at the end of the session for stray miniatures. This underlies the importance of order in the workshop and gives to students a rotating leadership opportunity.
- There is an important caveat: sometimes a student requests that a tray be left intact in order to extend and modify it in the next session. Comply if possible. The lid of the container is placed over the world and it is stored until the student returns.

## Role of teacher

It is not too much to say that the classroom must be reinvented as nest, stronghold, cradle, cave, shelter, rampart, and refuge.

- Be aware that it is the teacher who sets the atmosphere.
- Be the silent, non-judgmental witness to the work of the students, affirming their freedom to create. Set boundaries around the process by quietly insisting on the rules of silence and no trading of miniatures.
- Avoid any impulse to interpret sand pictures.
- Be responsive to needs of individual students.
    - Some kindergarten students need to point out what they have made as their world is in process. Waiting to share the entire world is too difficult. Be available to hear their explanations.
    - At the outset, some children are uncomfortable with the narrative form. Jackson, for example, struggling with a language disability, at first was uncomfortable with imaginative worlds. Instead, he built elaborate bridges and vehicles. His written records were procedures, not narratives. He spent days replicating the solar system in his sandtray. Liz Hollands, in her role as educational assistant, honoured his need to create factual content in the tray, helping him research and read abundant informational text on the solar system. The aim was to provide him with a vehicle for expression. His frequent tantrums lessened in number and intensity as he was given freedom to work on the projects he chose. After about three months of focus on facts and information, he felt confident to produce an imaginary world in the tray and to tell its story. It was a tale about the mayor of a town, named Mayor Jackson.
    - Sometimes a student requests a miniature that is of particular importance in his series of sand pictures, but that is contained that day in another bag. If it is possible without untoward disruption, meet that student's request for the miniature.

- Record keeping:
    - Photograph the completed world. Store the photographs on individual student computer drives. This creates a student portfolio of the sand picture series which students can access in order to create a movie version of their stories with narration and to which they can refer as a stimulus to storywriting in the regular class. (See Chapters 4 and 6.)
    - The student portfolio means that student and teacher can track the progression of themes, content, and organization in the sandworld series.
    - The care with which the teacher tracks and stores the sandworld pictures speaks to students about how they are valued.
    - The sandtray world is not something to be marked or evaluated. Track engagement and behaviour by means of observation and anecdotal records.
    - Distribute 1–10 rating scales, surveys, and self-reflections on attitude and interest at the outset of the sandtray experience and at the end of term. Address specifics such as school engagement, enjoyment, focus, and behaviour. If you are a resource teacher offering the sandplay within a special education resource withdrawal setting, give the same rating scale and survey to the student's classroom teacher.

# VIOLENCE IN SANDWORLDS

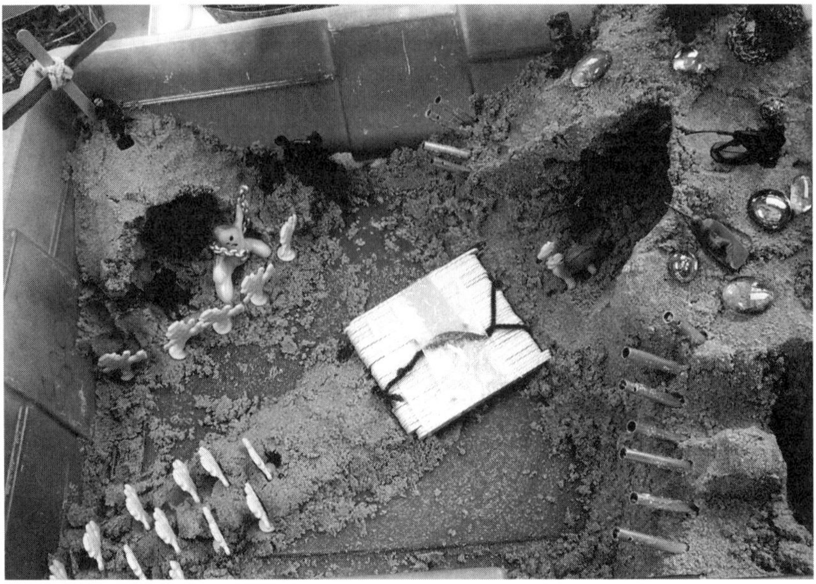

*Figure 3.2 World of conflict and impending struggle*

'It smells like rotting corpses as the shots are fired at us' (Figure 3.2). A builder is telling the story of his sandworld recently in a group conference of boys. His words are met with low whistles and a chorus of 'Wow!' and 'Right on!'

'That's a *good* one!' someone adds admiringly.

Battle, struggle, dissolution, and danger are recurring scenes in sandworlds, showing up most commonly in the trays of boys. Is the prevalence of violence in boys' creative work because violence is the acceptable ethos among them? Because these are the circumstances in which they bond? Because therein lies social capital? (See Fletcher 2006; Pollack 1998.) We can guess that these are all contributing factors. In addition, however, it is important to note that in the trajectory of a sandtray series, struggle constitutes a necessary phase.

Various writers refer to the process of sandplay as cycling through stages of chaos, struggle, and resolution (Allan and Brown 1993; Bradway *et al.* 1990; Kalff 1980). 'Chaos' stage trays look just like the name would imply: a conglomeration of objects randomly flooding the sand. When the scene begins to show organized battles – initially without a winner or with the 'bad guys' winning – the trays can be said to be in the stage of 'Struggle' (Figure 3.2). Gradually, according to Allan, the adversaries are not killed, but imprisoned, and a hero emerges who wins over evil. 'Resolution' stage trays emerge when order is restored and a balance is evident. However, sandtray scenes do not usually progress from one stage to the next in a straight line; instead, they often fluctuate between stages. This three-stage formulation, then, calls for fighting and violence as necessary in the progression from chaos to resolution.

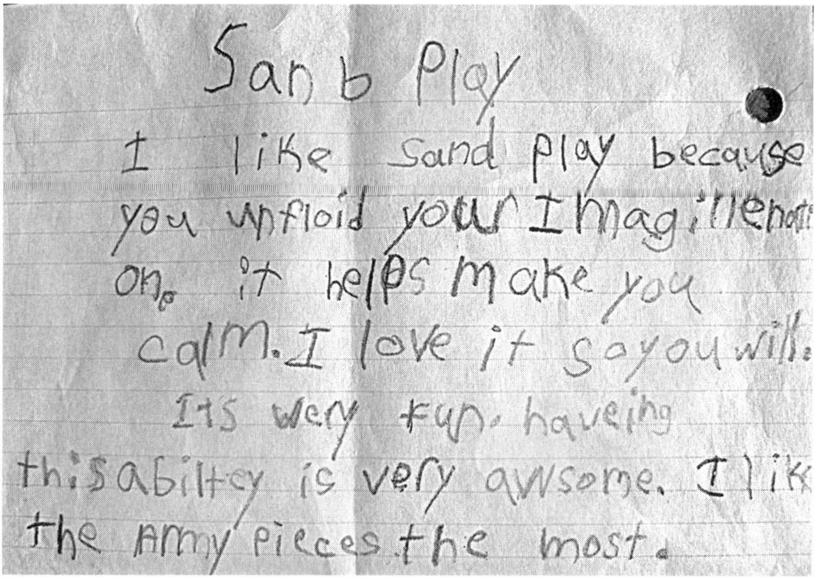
Sanb Play
I like sand play because
you unfloid your Imagillenati
on. it helps make you
calm. I love it so you will.
Its wery fun. haveing
thisabiltey is very awsome. I lik
the Army pieces the most.

*Figure 3.3 'I like the army pieces the most'*

In the testimonial about his sandplay experience (Figure 3.3), a student makes two salient observations: 'It makes me calm' and 'I like the army pieces the most.' At first glance, it seems counterintuitive that a feeling of calm runs alongside the conflict suggested by army pieces. My sense, though, is that his calm is in fact due to the inclusion of the army pieces. Within the safe context of the tray he is free to find expression for dispute, tension, discord, and argument, to face issues of power and danger, to meet these, and to sort them out. The end result is a feeling of calm.

## EXAMPLES OF SANDWORLD SERIES

In sandtray work each student has an individual approach to the stuff of creation. Some organize the figures first; others begin by setting vegetation and topography; some arrive to the workshop with a plan already envisioned for their world and set about to find the figures needed; others are seemingly random in their choices. Some builders have difficulty keeping their world contained within the sandtray and want to expand their building territory. Some build perfunctorily because their felt desire is to share the story as soon as possible, learning only over weeks to extend and deepen the building experience. The sandtray series of Tamare, Garthe, and Ellie, reported below, demonstrate that growth in organization of the sandtray is reflected and accompanied by growth in social, emotional, and academic areas.

### Tamare: Learning containment

At first, Tamare, a Grade 2 (age seven) student, scattered sand out of her tray as if splashing water at the swimming pool. Her desk and floor space were gritty. She balked at building her world within the four walls of the tray. She spread out her territory to encompass the floor and bookshelf nearby. Her sandworlds were chaotic (Figure 3.4).

In a striking parallel, Tamare lacked awareness of boundaries in both her social and academic life. Socially, Tamare intruded into the personal and psychological space of her peers. Her ability to sustain attention was limited. It was only infrequently and with great effort that she was able to curb her curiosity about what her nearest classmate was building. Academically, she struggled with the task of organizing her written work, unaware that certain letters consistently represented certain sounds, that spaces were needed between words, that words were formed between lines.

Containing the sand and limiting her world to the tray during the building segment; listening without interruption during the sharing; spacing words and placing letters on the line while writing – all would require learning to notice and work with physical limits and boundaries. All would require containment.

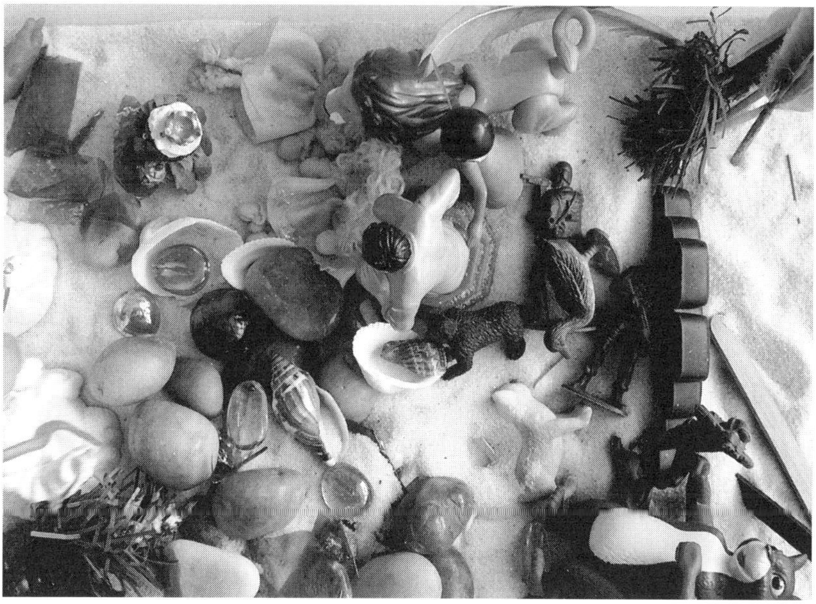

*Figure 3.4 Chaos: Tamare's early world*

Tamare participated in seven months of a daily sandtray narrative workshop comprising a group of 12 students with teacher and assistant. By end-of-year she had made significant progress in listening with attention to her partner's story, observing appropriate boundaries while building, and attending to letter formation and spacing. My sense was that the progress Tamare made in the areas of academics and social interaction was related to the progress she made in observing the boundaries of the sandtray.

In her penultimate tray, Tamare placed a container in which, she writes, are three gifts from three friends: a candle from the friend she names Sara, a flower from a boy she calls Max, and a round Frisbee from one she names Cristal. Like her organized sandworld, the printed words of her story are carefully spaced and placed on the line. Her story is titled 'The Vase' (Figure 3.5). Here, appropriately, in the shape of the vase is a container within the larger container of the tray. The three gifts it holds are candlelight, a living flower, and the contours of a circle.

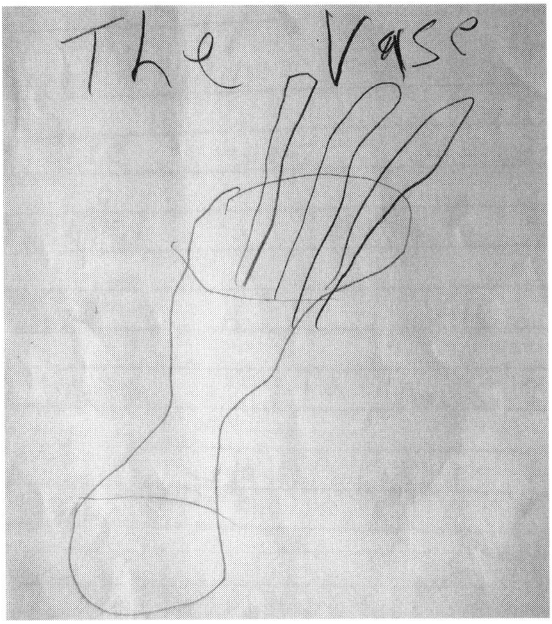


*Figure 3.5 The Vase: Cover page for Tamare's end-of-year story*

## Garthe: Separating water from land

Garthe was a seven-year-old who worked in a before-school sandtray group of two students. At the outset of his sandtray sessions he was struggling with angry outbursts. His drawing of an erupting volcano illustrates what he was feeling (Figure 3.6). The water of his early sandworlds flooded the dry land. During the building of his series of worlds, a gradual separation of water from land paralleled his working out of how to cope with emotions that had been overwhelming him.

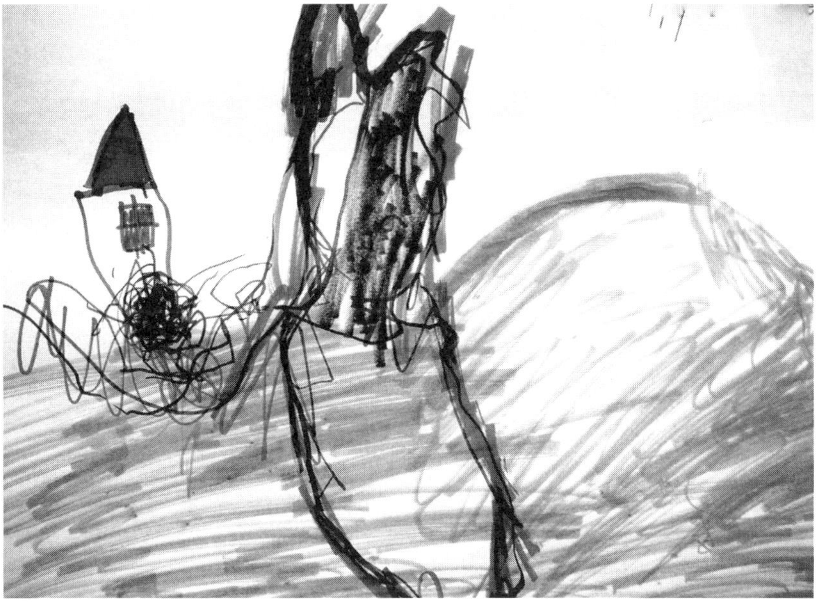

*Figure 3.6 Volcano*

Garthe flooded his initial series of trays with water, as seen in Figure 3.7.

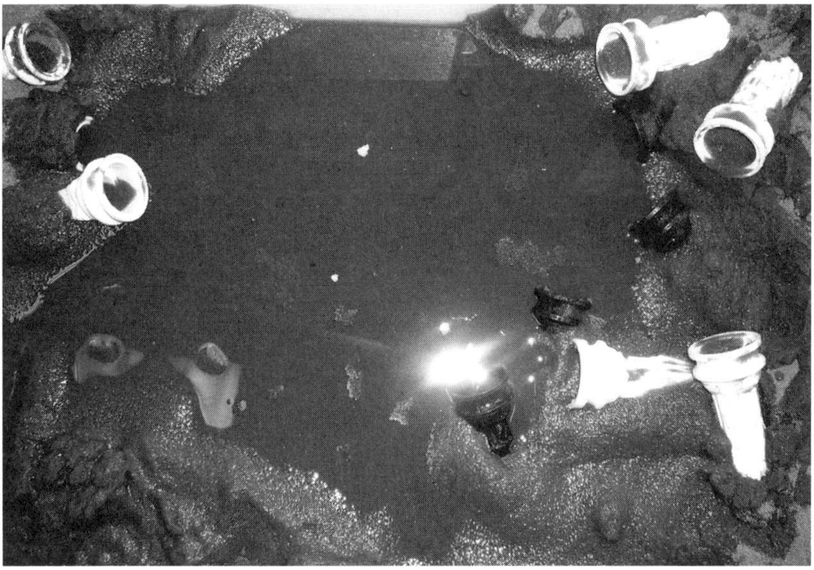

*Figure 3.7 Flooding*

Over a number of months, Garthe separated out the water from the land. He built boats. At first, houses were half submerged. With successive trays, the houses began to find footing on an island, as seen in Figure 3.8.

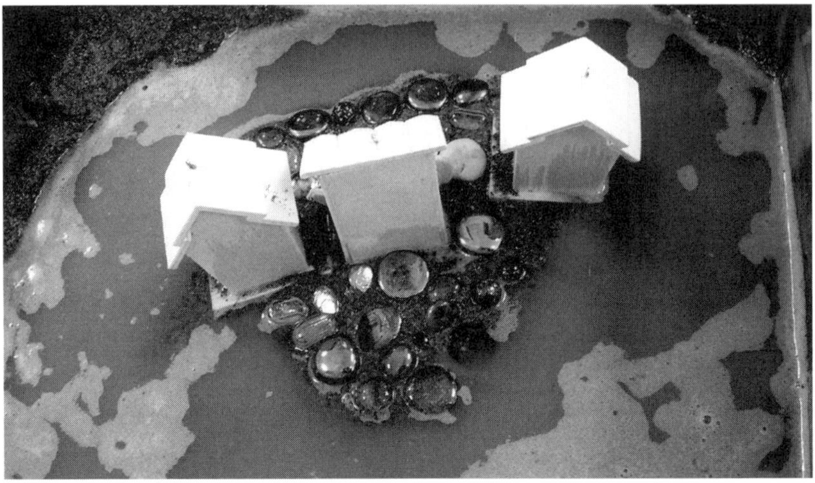

*Figure 3.8 Water separating from land*

The house in Figure 3.9 is now on firm footing on an island surrounded by what Garthe called 'the blue jewels'.

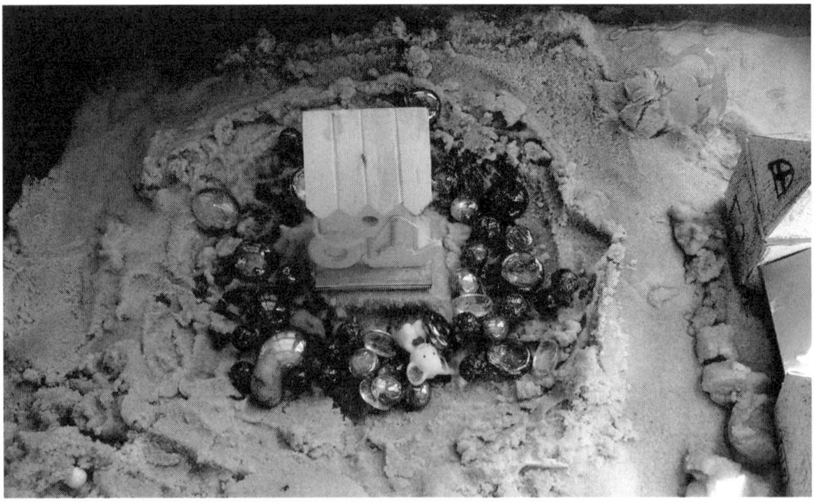

*Figure 3.9 Island*

Here, in Figure 3.10, is Garthe's mandala-like drawing of the island world of the sandtray of Figure 3.9. Notice the smiling sunshine in the upper left corner.

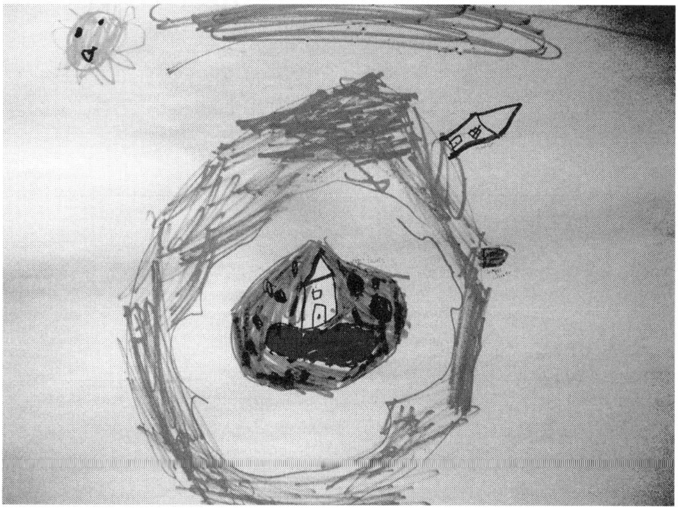

*Figure 3.10 Drawing of island*

## Ellie: Learning organization

The junior kindergarten student, Ellie, showed progress with the physical organization of the objects in the tray, paralleling an increased clarity in her formulation of oral language. Ellie's ability to tell the story about her worlds improved along the same trajectory as her ability to organize the worlds themselves, the clarity of her spoken expression growing apace with the physical intelligibility of her trays. It leads me to wonder whether there is a reciprocal development between expressive language organization and visual organization.

Initially, Ellie's speech was very difficult to understand. Her language lacked basic grammatical markers. A formal speech and language assessment provided recommendations upon which her individual education plan learning expectations were based. These included following two-part directions containing terms such as 'before', 'after', 'last', 'in', 'on', 'under', 'beside'; asking and answering 'wh' questions, and increasing the use of the irregular past tense.

Ellie's initial sandtrays were chaotic as we see in the scene of Figure 3.11: overturned cars, fence rails in piles, figures buried by the random acts of popsicle (lolly) sticks. She uses every figure available to her in that tray. Her story was 'the cat is going to the bathroom'.

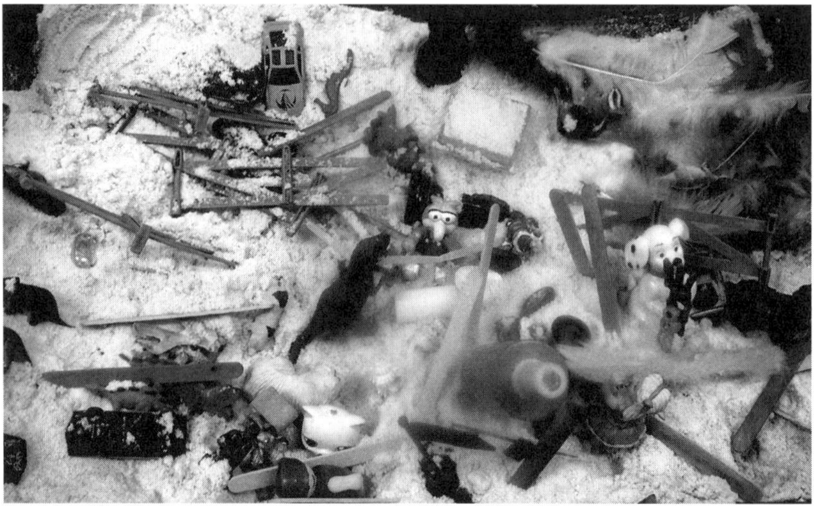

*Figure 3.11 Ellie's first tray*

After six weeks of a small group sandtray storymaking workshop twice weekly, Ellie was using fences to delineate specific parts of the world (Figure 3.12). Three separate areas define space for separate figures. There is a seahorse inside a fenced-in area, a dinosaur behind a barrier that is held up at one end by a dog, a cat inside a contained area on a square, and finally a girl inside what Ellie called a 'room', at the base of a flag. All the objects in this tray are placed with careful deliberation and the organization appears in striking contrast to the randomness of the initial tray.

Ellie's story about the tray pictured in Figure 3.12 delineated characters, setting, problem, and solution. The organization of her language had increased in parallel development with increased visual organization of her sandworld. The story was as follows:

> Pointing to the girl, Ellie said, ''Cause she's sleeping. She's tired. That's her room.'

Pointing to the cat on the square, Ellie said, 'That's the cat. That's her room. She's so bad she always got gum on her tail.'

She repeated: 'That girl is sleeping. That's her room.'

Next Ellie articulated a plot problem. 'Dinosaur is going to bite the girl. She is going to bite her castle.' Finally, Ellie showed the solution to the problem: 'The dinosaur won't get her because her mommy (the dog) is there.'

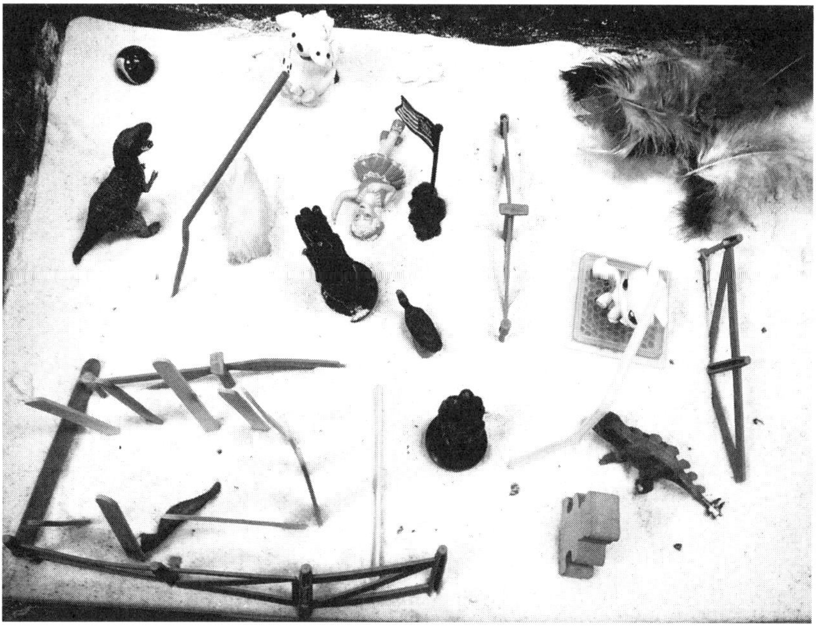

*Figure 3.12 Ellie's tray, six weeks later*

## STEALING AND BREAKING OF FIGURINES: SUGGESTIONS FOR TROUBLESHOOTING

For some children, the glitter of a dollar store ring or the niftiness of a small car is irresistibly beguiling. Although our school sandplay collections comprise of inexpensive items, it is not the monetary value that is at issue with stealing or breakage. Rather, these troublesome acts provide teachable moments about respect for classroom property and about trust.

1. *Declare a boundary* around the collection. Set it at the outset. In the same way that we instruct sandplayers not to put their hands in the worlds of their classmates or disturb what another has created, we put boundaries around the class collection of miniatures. The miniatures are for the children, we tell them, but for use in this one setting at this one time. In this way, we model to our students how they can put boundaries around their own personal belongings, and respect the belongings of others.

2. *Avoid two extremes*, neither saddling a student with a burden of guilt nor ignoring an incident, thereby inuring a student to wrongdoing. If stealing or deliberate breakage happens, confront it in a simple, matter-of-fact way: the sandplay miniatures belong in the sandplay room and need to stay there, be cared for, and not damaged. If called for in the particular circumstance, a student may need to make amends. Much depends upon the age of the child and the particular situation.

3. *Co-create a story*. A story gives distance that provides emotional safety. Although children's storybooks are one tool to use to forge a safe space in which to confront these difficult topics, making up a story means that you can tailor the problem and resolution to the specific situation faced in the classroom. In composing a co-created story, the teacher can involve the children in problem-solving the issue at hand. Use the following guidelines:

    - Begin the story by creating characters and setting with one or two lively details:
      *Once upon a time there was a little elephant named Bertha. She lived with all her friends in the savanna. She had very big ears and a long snuffly nose. What she liked to do above all else was to make worlds in a tray.*

    - Add the complicating problem, the problem at hand in the classroom – perhaps stealing or destruction of miniatures:
      *There were so many beautiful things in the sandtray place in the savanna, but one day, one thing above all stood out for her. It was*

*a green snake with jeweled eyes. Bertha desperately wanted it. She imagined how much fun it would be to take it out at recess. But it belonged to the play collection. How hard that was for her! It was not her snake but she wanted it. She thought and thought and thought about it. Then one day, she tried to sneak it away.*

(Alternatively, she might be angry and she broke it, or she might hide it so no one could find it.)

- Invite the children to participate in creating the resolution: *Then she felt so bad that she... What do you think she did, children? What do you think she could do? What would you advise her to do?*

  (Alternatively, the elephant might decide to tell her teacher how badly she wanted the toy and *what do you think the teacher said to her?*)

- A story provides a non-confrontational way to air the topic of temptation or wrongdoing.
- Articulation of the feelings of the main character serves to remove a sense of isolation and helplessness from the child who is struggling with the problem.
- The children themselves will come up with ideas of how to help the character that is facing such an issue and how the story problem could be resolved.
- After the group problem-solving experience in the safe space of the co-created story, you have a common language with which to talk about stealing or breakage, one that you and your students have developed together.
- On the feeling and imaginative level, you have developed the student's ownership of responsibility for care of the classroom materials.

## Chapter 4

# TELLING

*'My favourite part is that we get to explain it to the whole group.'*

– Monty, Grade 6 (age 11)

*'I have a great idea in my head but as soon as I put it into words I have trouble explaining it. I lose it when I try to tell it.'*

– Joel, Grade 5 (age ten)

*'The good thing about telling: it is good to tell because if you mess up you just fix it.'*

– Maria, Grade 4 (age nine)

The sandworld is complete. Through the light-heartedness of play, the topography has been prepared, the sand shaped or molded into hills, plains, lakes, chasms, rivers, ramparts, caves, towers. Vegetation has been added, perhaps dwelling places, and the terrain further defined with rocks, sticks, and feathers. The characters that inhabit the world have been chosen and placed not with conscious deliberation but in answer to some playful impulse or attraction. They may be standing or partially buried or poised to run or entrapped in an enclosure or playing. A tension or dialogue has emerged between the figures in the world by reason of their placement in relation to each other. In its completion, the whole scene may show a sense of flow or disruption, of emptiness or fullness, of peace or conflict, of order or chaos (Weinberg 2007, p.150). We might say that the sand picture intimates characters, setting, problem, and solution.

Characters, setting, problem, and solution – these are elements of narrative structure! And it is a narrative that the students are now asked to tell. 'Tell the story of your world to your partner,' we instruct them. They are invited to put language to the world, construct the narrative, and tell it to others.

There is an answering impulse in the student – a desire to share, to communicate the richness of the inner story that has engrossed them as they played. Builders invariably are eager to share their world: as 11-year-old Monty said, 'My favourite part is that we get to explain it to the whole group.' In sharing, students become practitioners of an essential art, the art of making meaning through making story. 'We are the meaning makers, every one of us: children, parents, and teachers. To try to make sense. To construct stories. And to share them with others in speech and in writing is an essential part of being human' (Wells 1986, p.222).

Some children build in meditative silence, choosing a series of miniatures and placing them in the tray, with no outer sign of inner commentary. Other children whisper a story to themselves using a private language – a kind of inner, condensed speech, complete with sound track, dialogue, and action – a story that seems to bubble up, called forth from the figures, the surrounding silence, and the child's imagination. Regardless of building style, the child builder-turned-teller is now required to construct a framework of meaning with words. Inner speech will become outer speech, a deliberate, organized mode that will make sense to a listener. The shorthand leaps of play have to be explained, the parameters of the world described.

## FROM BUILDING TO TELLING: WHAT IS GOING ON?

Joel is a student in Grade 5 (age ten) who builds intriguing worlds full of danger and excitement and with an element of the numinous. According to Joel, it is not easy to make the transition from building to telling. One morning he reflects on this as he shares his experience: 'I have a great idea in my head but as soon as I put it into words I have trouble explaining it,' he says. 'I lose it when I try to tell it.' In an observation that sounds very much like Joel's, White (1980) writes, 'Narrative might well be considered the solution to a problem of general concern, namely, the problem of translating knowing into telling' (cited in Hudson and Shapiro 1991, p.89).

What happens when the knower becomes the teller? What are the paths whereby inner thoughts, ideas, and images become communicated to another person? These are heady questions and for philosophers, linguists, and psychologists. However, because right here in the schoolroom, worldmakers-turned-storytellers such as Joel are grappling with the same questions, let's consider them briefly. At the very least we can say that when the builder of the world tells her story:

- speaking and listening replace seeing
- thought that is undirected is organized and communicated outwardly
- a world is constructed through the use of words.

## Seeing is replaced by speaking and listening

Vygotsky (1934/1986) reflects that what we conceive of as one thought can be expressed only by putting it into many separate, consecutive units of speech. He writes, 'A thought may be compared to a cloud shedding a shower of words... In [the speaker's] mind the whole thought is present at once, but in speech it has to be developed successively' (p.251). Like a thought, the sand picture is a unit. It stands alone in its entirety, mute and expressive to the beholder's eye. Perhaps in one corner of the tray, a dragon is rising protectively over a brown dog, which is holding a bone at the entrance to a cave that is situated beside a lake. The largeness of the towering dragon, the darkness of the cave, the dog's nondescript fur, and the blueness of the lake – all this can be taken in, in a single instant, by the one looking at the tray. 'A picture is worth a thousand words', the saying goes. What the eye grasps in a moment the ear understands only over many minutes, word by successive word. The teller requires time and a deliberate use of language, as what has been formed as a sand picture is communicated with speech.

## 'Undirected thought' is communicated

Reflect for a moment on the kind of thinking that you do when you are engaged in a reverie or daydream; then contrast it with the kind of thinking you do when you are explaining to someone an insight that you have acquired or an incident you have experienced. You might say that the first kind of thinking uses images; the second uses words. In his essay 'The Language and Thought of the Child', Piaget (1923/1977) describes two distinct modes of thinking. One he labels 'directed' or conscious; the other 'undirected' or unconscious. 'Directed thought' is oriented to outer reality, can be judged either true or false, is logical, and is guided by the need to communicate. It is the thinking required in explaining the insight or recounting the incident. By contrast, 'undirected thought' is not adapted to outer reality, but creates its own world of imagination; it communicates through images and connects to symbols. It is the thought of the reverie and daydream. 'Undirected thought' is an intuitive, syncretistic, personal, imagistic, leaping kind of thought.

Take the boat, for example. To 'directed thought' the boat is a tangible object. Craftsmen study and perfect its manufacture and it floats because of the physics of buoyancy. A student composition about the boat might be submitted as a science fair project on flotation or a history report on the *Mayflower*. By contrast, to 'undirected thought' the boat might be an ark of safety, making feasible a journey over water, a liminal space between earthly time and watery eternity, a womb or cradle of psychological birth. Writing that comes out of 'undirected thought' might sound as follows: *The boat is more coracle than ship, more cradle than coracle. The sail is down. The pilot surrenders to the currents and the waves, waiting. Waiting, as the boat dips and recovers, dips and recovers.*

Piaget concludes:

> The mere fact, then, of telling one's thought, of telling it to others, or of keeping silence and telling only to oneself must be of enormous importance to the fundamental structure and functioning of thought in general, and of child logic in particular. (p.86)

Because the sandplayer builds a world through play and reverie, Piaget's 'undirected thought' might be considered a template for understanding the kind of thinking processes involved during building. Children build in a freewheeling, stream-of-consciousness kind of activity, often repeating mythical themes in the tray. The sandtray is the 'undirected thought' of the child, shown and shaped in the sand. The step of relaying in words the images of the imaginative world of the sandplay is an important leap. The two modes of 'undirected' and 'directed' thought are not opposed; rather, they meet together in the telling of story, the 'undirected' thought acting as a wellspring of ideas and images for it. Because, as Neumann writes, the child at play has been embedded 'in the magical-mythical symbol-world' (1988, p.70), the language of story, myth, and symbol is eminently suited to the telling.

### A secondary world is constructed

The builder-turned-teller becomes the maker of what Tolkien calls a 'Secondary World'. The storyteller creates a world into which a listener can enter, suspending engagement in the business of his own life in order to do so:

> What really happens is that the story-maker proves a successful 'sub-creator.' He makes a Secondary World which your mind can enter. Inside it, what he relates is 'true': it accords with the laws of that world. You therefore believe it, while you are, as it were, inside. (1964, p.36)

This is the art of storytelling at its most realized, and the goal to which we invite our students. Day after day, using the support of the sand picture in varying degrees, as students tell the stories of a succession of trays, they build proficiency with constructing 'secondary worlds'. The effect of this practice is that children realize what Gordon Wells described as 'the symbolic potential of language: its power to create possible and imaginary worlds through words' (1986, p.156).

## VARIETIES OF STORYTELLING: NAMING, DRAMATIZING, NARRATING

The language of story is distinct. It is sometimes called decontextualized language (Kaderavak and Sulzby 2000). It is unlike conversation and collaboration, in which the participants share dialogue or experience together and meanings are jointly constructed. Instead of pointing to the pot on the kitchen floor and saying to the playmate standing beside her, 'Look at the pot!' or noticing a frog and saying, 'Watch it jump!', the child who is telling someone *about* a remembered pot or an imagined frog has at her disposal only words to communicate the message. What is needed is not the single word 'Look!' but descriptive labels and verbs, not 'she' and 'it', but nouns and adjectives. In telling stories, children are in fact learning to use language that is essential to literacy. Not surprisingly, researchers have discovered that skill in using decontextualized language is a key predictor of literacy and school achievement (Nicolopoulou, McDowell, and Brockmeyer 2006). Storytelling may be seen as a stepping stone to literacy.

There are bridges for children learning to use decontextualized language of story. The sandtray is one such bridge. Like pictures in an illustrated storybook, a cartoon in a comic book, or the stage set in a drama, the sandtray provides a shared visual context between storyteller and listener. The world built in the sand, eloquent in its physicality, acts as a scaffold for the telling, supporting learners as they develop skill in using decontextualized language.

Storymakers use the support of the shared context to varying degrees. Some rely heavily upon the visual of the sandworld. At the other end of the continuum, the teller uses a picture in the sand as a jumping-off point for a fully developed narrative.[1] Types of sandtray narratives can be categorized in terms of the use the teller makes of the sandtray – naming, dramatizing, and narrating.

- *Naming:* Naming-mode stories rely heavily upon the tray. The storyteller points to specific objects within the sandworld and tells the listener what they are, identifying them and perhaps

1 The researchers, Stadler and Ward (2005), similarly argue that oral storytelling progresses from a hodgepodge of unrelated statements that describe or give labels, to a stage where there is an internal configuration that organizes the statements – first around a central topic, then with temporal sequence, then with the addition of character goals and causality. The final evolution of the story, they propose, is seen in the narrative that has not only organization, but a central theme or moral and a developed plot. They called these stages, respectively, Labeling, Listing, Connecting, Sequencing, and Narrating.

pointing out their salient attributes. These stories sound like a salad of unrelated statements and, as the teller's language develops, like lists.

- *Dramatizing:* 'I don't know how the story goes if I don't do it with my hands. My body does the story.' Abel's words give us an eloquent description of the dramatizing mode. Stories in this category are told as dramas, narrated as the teller enacts the plot while moving the figures in the tray. The teller may not be able to predict the end of the story at the outset of the drama. The action in the sandtray supplements the words of the story; conversely, the words of the story comment on the action in the sandtray.
- *Narrating:* Narrating-category stories make use of the tray as a jumping-off point from which the narrator begins the tale and to which he can refer during the process of telling. This is a broad category in which the finished sandworld functions as a reference point. Tellers of stories in the narrating mode are developing facility with both structure and language of narrative.

Look at the hands of the storytellers. The hands of naming- and dramatizing-mode storytellers are in their sandtrays while they tell their stories. The trays are integral to the telling, providing indispensable context as the narrative is related. These narratives fall at the contextualized end of the storytelling spectrum. By comparison, stories in the narrating mode fall at the decontextualized end of the spectrum – an assertion corroborated by the hands of tellers of these stories, which are seldom in the tray. It is important to note that the three modalities of storymaking do not necessarily follow each other sequentially. Students spiral around the range of naming, dramatizing, and narrating, depending on the complexity of what they have to say. Furthermore, a particular story may use the support of the tray to various degrees as learners develop facility with the language of narrative.

## Naming mode: Stories that are told as labels

Naming-stories sound a bit like the finger play 'Here is the church / Here is the steeple / Open the door / There's all the people'. It is the barebones labeling, listing, and describing of the items that are physically pointed out. There is no organization that brings them into relationship. It is the language I use with my nine-month-old grandchild: 'mommy', 'dog', 'water', 'toes', 'bump'. It is the language of Adam in the creation story where he is brought 'every living creature to see what he would call them' (Genesis 2:4, NRSV 1989). It is the action whereby, Rumpelstiltskin-like, we gain power over what is, by speaking its name. It is the language that all sandplayers – children and adults alike – use some of the time.

In a kindergarten group, one student lists her characters: 'This is Cinderella. This is the kid. These are flags and bushes. This is my horsie. This is an airplane.' Another says: 'That is the snake. These are rocks. These are jewels. This is my basket.' Carmen, a student in Grade 2 (age seven) says, 'That's the house!' She pauses, looks up and adds in a voice full of import, 'And that's the guard.'

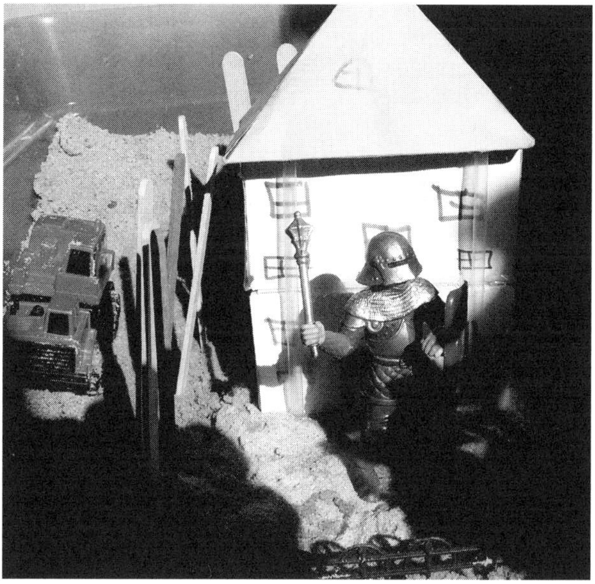

*Figure 4.1 Naming: Labels as signifiers of a layered story. 'That's the house,' says Carmen. 'And' (wide-eyed with emphasis) 'that's the guard.'*

At first blush, these lists of labels may not sound like narratives; however, they carry story within them. The play therapist Kestly (2010) refers us to the work of Damasio, a neuroscientist (1999), who argues that language is only a second step, a translation of what is at the core of our thinking – the core comprising of sensory-based images. Language gives us names for these images; it gives us labels. Labels bear resonance for the sandplayer; they hold a whole world of associations. Labels are not simply discrete identifications of objects. Rather, they are markers for the inner sensory-based images we have and contain layers of reference, emotion, history, experience, and memory. For the teenaged girl who placed a dragonfly in the tray and said, 'It is a dragonfly. I don't know why. I just put it there. One wing is broken', the dragonfly in the tray is resonating with the memory of dragonflies on the summer dock, a song she has heard about the dragonfly, an association she has with the fragile-looking power of the wings. In Carmen's case (see Figure 4.1), a house under siege recurred repeatedly one spring. It was later this year that her parents' marriage dissolved and the family reconfigured. The labeling of 'the guard' perhaps expresses the inner story of the powerful protector, the labeling of 'the house' the story of what is in danger.

### *Example of story told in naming mode*

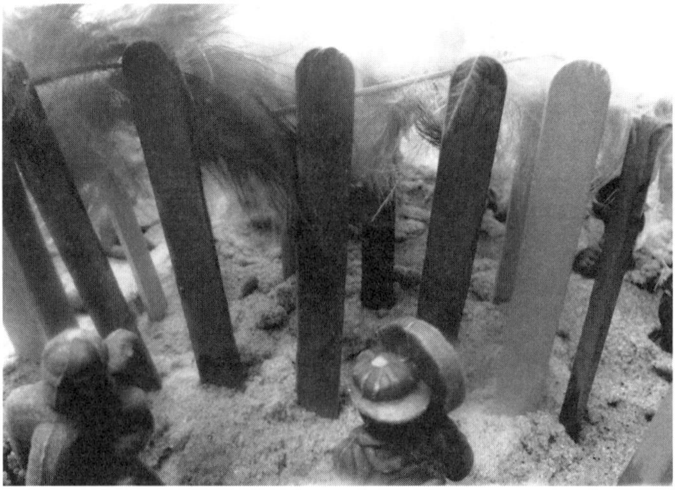

*Figure 4.2 The Never-Ending Maze*

In the example of a naming mode story told by a student in Grade 7 (age 12) about the world pictured in Figure 4.2, the elements of the sandworld and the actions of the characters are listed. The story is titled 'The Never-Ending Maze'.

## THE NEVER-ENDING MAZE

This is a never-ending maze. No way in. No way out. No start. No end. Some people have made their way in. I don't know how. I put these sticks everywhere. But some people have made their way in. For example, these people: they are researchers.

A little boy got lost because he was inside the ground. This guy with the phone is calling just to make sure there is no one in the maze. This one (*pointing*) has something in his ear. Because he is looking for sounds across the maze to make sure there is no one in the maze. I have this little guy in here (*pointing*). He got into the maze and he is calling the guys. So we have three guys looking for sound. No one was in the maze. Only what there was, was a baby boy. This is the animal area. The animals are on the outside of the maze.

Now this guy is looking for gold and he finds something. He is trying to look for more. He hasn't found any yet. He found the nugget, the gold fish, and the big gold nugget. And he found other things. A blue jewel. That is all he found so far.

Now this is the most interesting. See this box, it is actually a trap. If an animal goes on the outside, that alarm will go off and it will trap him. It will knock him out. I have another animal trap, for a little animal. So if this animal starts there, the trap will fall and trap it. On its head. I like the trap part. It is covered in feathers so it looks decorative. It is actually a trick. I put the feathers on.

Now we don't know what is going to happen. Because now, actually, there are people in it. Yes, now there are people in it. We don't know what is going to happen. But here is a hint: my next world is going to be where these guys are going to make it into a real maze that really starts and really ends. Because the man that made the maze that never started, he died. So these guys are going to take over!

In the story of the never-ending maze, the setting is described masterfully (*no way in, no way out*). The problem in the story is implied in the setting – the never-ending maze. The overarching feeling is that of lostness and blockage. There is a man mining for treasure, researchers calling into the maze, animals which are trapped through the deceptive feathers. The relationships between the characters in various parts of the worlds are not clearly revealed. There is a sense of narrative but the plot is not articulated overtly; rather, it is implied through the labeling. The solution to the problem in this story, we are told, has already happened; almost as if by articulating the problem, it was eradicated, for *the man who made the maze died*. That the problem has been solved will be evident in the next world in which the setting will be a maze that has both entrance and exit.

## Dramatizing mode: Stories that are told as theatre

In dramatizing mode, the finished sandworld provides the opening setting for a story. With the witnessing listener present, the teller modifies the world while chronicling the action. He might begin to move the car that is parked in the cave he had formed in the sandtray, for example, and move it around a track, and then add another car and embark upon a blow-by-blow description of a race. What follows is a running commentary on the movements in the sandworld, as well as a running dialogue between the characters. The plot is enacted; the figures are props; the sandplay is a drama; the listener is a spectator. This is distinct from naming mode because the child actively engages with the world, manipulating the figures, as he describes what is happening.

Piaget identifies a mode of speech in which the child talks aloud to herself in front of others. He names this a 'collective monologue' (1923/1977, p.74). The term helps us understand what is happening in dramatizing-mode stories because of the dual nature of the stories in that mode. Dramatizing-category stories sound like monologues; however, because the child is aware of the witness at the same time as she is speaking, the monologues are shared.

Because the physical gestures accompany the child's verbalization, supplementing the description of the action, much does not have to be articulated and the linguistic task is not as onerous. The characters and their movements speak for themselves. In fact, dramatizing-mode stories most clearly demonstrate the link between thought and action. They show thought being informed and developed by the movement in the sand. The sand shows what cannot be stated; the words state what cannot be shown. There is a sense of forward movement from problem to resolution in these stories, a temporal sequence, and sometimes an organization around a central topic, and demonstration of cause and effect.

### *Example of story told in dramatizing mode*

The following story is a dramatizing-mode narrative told by 12-year-old Kaleb about a wizard (shown in Figure 4.3) who dares to ask the forbidden question 'Where did you come from?' and, in the end, is able to return all the inhabitants of the world to their individual homes. Notice that the story begins in the past tense and moves into the present, the plot unfolding in front of our eyes. The teller relies heavily upon demonstrating the characters' actions by moving the characters as he speaks. In the example recorded below, the teller's actions are noted in italics. The asides, that give explanation about the plot to the audience, are noted in bold.

#### THE WIZARD AND THE TIME CAPSULE

*Glass pyramid is placed in the centre of the world, then a wizard and a flashlight.*

**Aside: The glass pyramid is a time capsule.**

*Back then a Wizard that wanted to be creative made a time capsule.*

*God was mad, took a shard (sea shell) and put it in front of the light. The shard there meant the people could not get back to their own home universe. (Student places shell/shard in front of the flashlight.)*

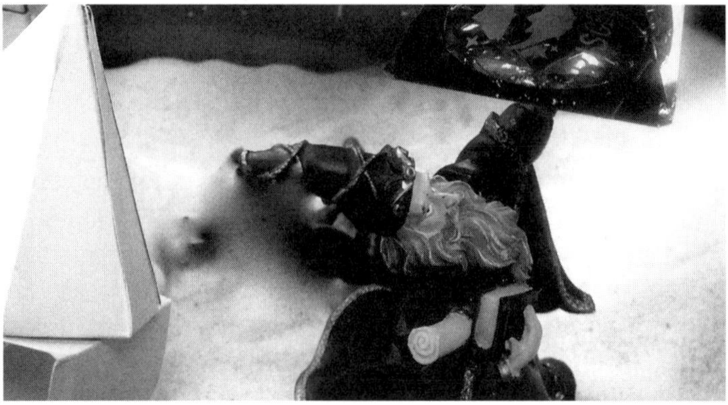

*Figure 4.3 Dramatizing-mode story: The Wizard and the Time Capsule*

The Wizard was the only one who asked questions. So he got badly beaten.

First the Wizard went to the police *(Adds the policeman.)*: 'Where did you come from?'

BOOM! The police knocks him out. *(Enacts policeman knocking down Wizard with a flourish and sound effects.)*

Then to the soldier: 'Where did you come from?' *(Moves the Wizard to face the soldier.)*

BOOM! The soldier knocks him out. *(Enacts soldier knocking down Wizard, Wizard making several attempts to retaliate, to no avail.)*

Then to the plane driver: *(Moves the Wizard to face the pilot.)* **Aside to audience: The plane driver lives in a water capsule, in a ship.** 'Where did you come from?' *(Tilts Wizard in a questioning posture.)* BOOM! The plane driver knocks him out. *(Enacts plane driver knocking down Wizard. Again Wizard is shown to put up a protracted fight.)*

Then to the Dragon: 'Where did you come from?' *(A violent battle is enacted between the Wizard and the Dragon, and the Wizard wins.)*

The Wizard wins over the Dragon! Since the Dragon was the keeper of the shard, the Wizard can now take the Dragon out into his own universe.

He took the Dragon into his own universe. *(Enacts the Dragon's removal.)*

Then the Wizard grabs the shard! All the inhabitants go home to their own universes!

## Narrating mode: Stories that are told as tales

Narrating mode refers to a broad category, distinguished by the teller's use of the sandtray. Rather than using the tray as a picture, its contents being listed, as in naming-mode stories, the teller attempts to link the various elements of the world to each other with causal connections as well as to incorporate elements of plot development. Rather than using the tray as the opening setting that is physically manipulated during the telling, as in dramatizing-stories, the tray is a jumping-off point or reference for the story. Because words alone carry the telling, narrating is sandtray storytelling in its most challenging mode. It requires decontextualized language.

Narrative organizes thoughts and content into a plan that incorporates characters, setting, problem, and solution (sometimes called the story's *macrostructure*) and depends upon the constructing and monitoring of meaning on a word and sentence level (sometimes called the story's *microstructure*) (Justice *et al.* 2006, p.178). Structure without lively language is dull and pedantic; words without the organization of a larger story structure leave the listener amused but not engaged. Tellers of stories in the narrating mode are developing facility with both structure and language of narrative.

Narrating mode encompasses a large territory along a continuum of competence. Stories manifest a wide variation, from beginning attempts that sound like plot outlines to mature stories in which the language is rich with description, the goals of characters embedded in the action, the plot told in past tense and moving towards a high point and resolution, the beginning, middle, and end in a cohesive flow. The following stories told by students from kindergarten to Grade 6 (age 11) demonstrate the wide continuum within the narrating mode.

### *Examples of narrating mode stories*

#### Example 1: 'The Dragon Guard'

A student in Grade 4 (age nine) articulates characters, problem, and solution in this tale of the scene shown in Figure 4.4. There is causality and linking between characters. The story is told with a mixture of past, present, and future tenses. In its entirety it sounds like a plot outline or summary with a final resolution in the dragon sacrifice.

## THE DRAGON GUARD

The bad guys found out about the treasure because they heard stuff at night. The good guys at night heard the sound of sharpening things. So the good guys are trying to save their treasure around here. The guy with the handgun can summon the dragon. The dragon will guard all over the place. If the good guy gets shot, he has five minutes to summon the dragon. It is a Chinese dragon, a water dragon. (But any kind of dragon can walk on land.) The dragon is going to give his whole entire soul. He will die. The good guys get strong from his soul and put the bad guys underground.

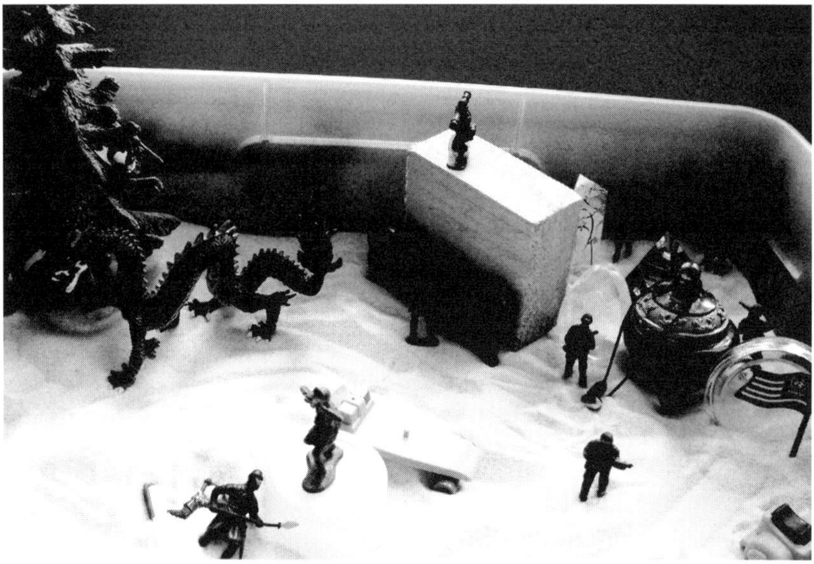

*Figure 4.4 Narrating mode – example 1: The Dragon Guard*

### Example 2: Untitled (Grade 6 (age 11) student)

Visuals for Kevin's untitled movie (Figure 4.5) were collected from various photographs of the sandtray, on which the camera would zoom in and away, giving a sense of motion while he narrated the action of the story. Kevin's narration sounds like an outline or précis of plot but contains descriptive language and some dramatic cadence. It is introduced with the moral lesson the teller wants to give to himself (and us). He makes use of a framework of characters, problem, and solution. The tense moves between past, present, and future.

## MOVIE TRANSCRIPT

There is a man, a dragon, and thousands of poisoned frogs. This is the story of one man who can control the dragon, but to have control of stuff is not always good. And sometimes if you have too much power, you will abuse it.

This man is digging a hole for the dragon to live in. But if he digs too deep, poison dart problems will start to come out at him. And then, if he gets poisoned by them, he will die a terrible death – a terrible, terrible death.

The guy dug too deep and the spiders and insects are trying to kill him. But he also went near a dinosaur's nest for her eggs. And now the dinosaur is really mad at him and might actually kill him by the end.

If you are wondering what that white thing is, it is a volcano that can erupt at any time. Here is the close-up of the man trying to get out of the hole. The man is trying to get out of the hole. There is the spider trying to kill him by biting his neck and there is a wasp and a lot of arachnids and frogs are coming all around him.

Five hours later: The man is still trying to get out. But there's more frogs reproducing like rabbits.

Boom! The volcano erupted! The spiders and frogs are trying to get away because they don't like the noise. The bee can stand it but it won't sting him because of the lava that is about to hit him. Luckily the volcano erupted right beside him and it is hitting all the rocks but it won't hit him. It hit all the rocks instead. And that's my story. Thanks for watching!

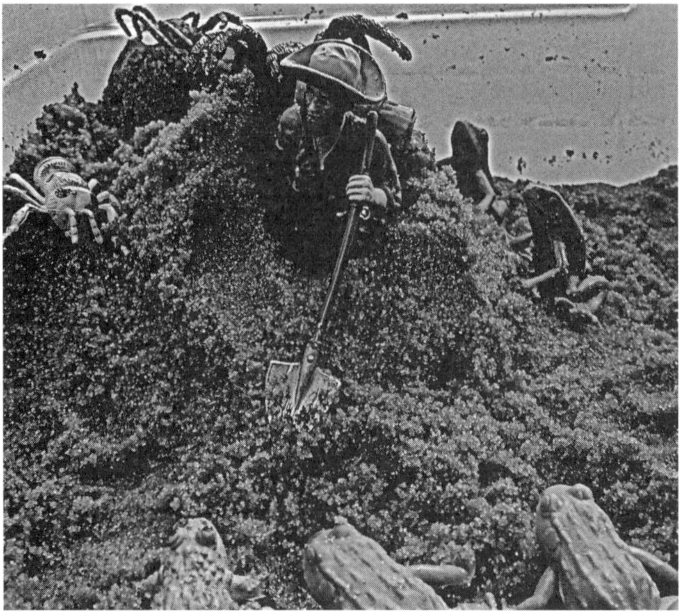

*Figure 4.5 Narrating mode – example 2: 'The close-up of the man trying to get out of the hole'*

### Example 3: Kindergarten stories

The following stories were told by two four-year-olds. There is complication in the action, a connection between the players in the tray, a problem stated. There are no descriptors. The problem and the conflict are stated in the future tense; the resolution is unknown.

#### JESS'S STORY

The king is in there. The guy on the bike wants to knock the castle down and live in it. He is going to go in there. And the dog will *try* to get him out.

#### AMY'S STORY

Strawberry Shortcake is sitting under the tree. The snowmen are trying to attack her. They are going to try to take her. They are going to put Strawberry Shortcake in the water.

## Example 4: 'The Greedy Giant'

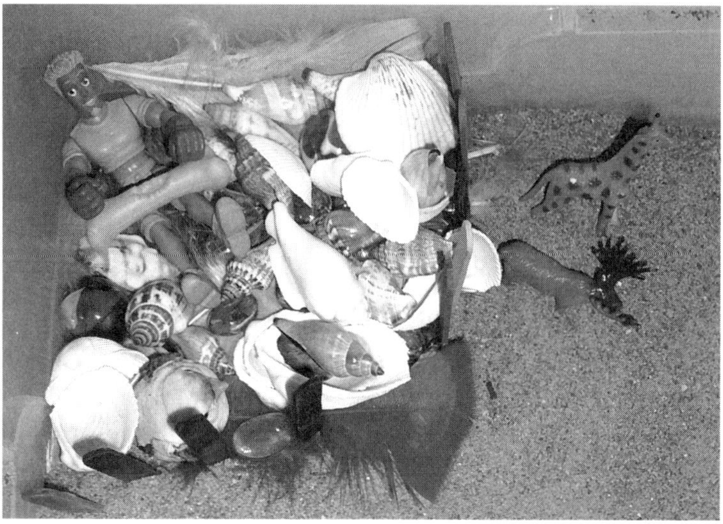

*Figure 4.6 Narrating mode – example 4: Greedy giant among his possessions*

In this example of the told story of a ten-year-old student, the elements of characters, setting, problem, and (pending) solution are articulated. The language in this story is well structured and approaches the poetic at times. The tense vacillates between present and future. There is a stated relationship between the various players and elements in the sandworld although the story seems to be divided into two segments: the first focusing on the greedy giant (who is shown in the detail of Figure 4.6) and the second on the conflict between the gods. At the end of the story there is a sense of suspended animation in the absence of a resolution between the forces of the Underworld and Overworld.

### THE GREEDY GIANT

The greedy giant only ever wants things. He feels everyone's things are meant to be his.

The three racers are racing to see which one will confront the giant and tell him to give all their things back. The loser will have to confront the giant. They all try to race across but there is a broken bridge and so they cannot finish the race. They decide to leave the giant until he dies. *THEN they shall take their things from him. If in the future any king or queen takes their things away, they will not be allowed.*

There are two guard animals guarding the greedy giant, a giraffe and a buck moose because the giant is not very smart and he thinks they are fierce. Beside the giant's guards is his daughter who does not do anything except stand there all day.

Here is the Shrine of Tawikia. It is a shrine to the god of Creation. The god can tell his children to do anything they want to the greedy giant to make sure the giant has a terrible life. The god of Creation has three children: NeiNei the water god, Tisha the land god, Tolaka the sky god. And there is the friendly scout, Talika. The greedy giant cannot go near the shrine.

Here across the water are the black gods. They are deadly enemies, the gods of the Underworld. They are the rivals of the gods of the Overworld. The horse figure is Daka, the Underworld creator. There is the Tower of Destruction, and the twin gods Vika, the god of hatred, and his twin, the god of war. The snake is the pet goddess of the Underworld. She is a semi-god. If her tail touches you, she can make you feel any feelings she wants you to feel. These dark gods are on the other side of the water. The creator of the Overworld made sure of this.

The creator of land split the land up into two places. The creator of the Underworld turned that land into a bare wasteland with few trees, burning with fire.

The gods of the Underworld want to get across the water. If they do, the Underworld god will defeat the creator god and force all his children into his army. But the water god keeps all the water slashing at their banks so they can't come near or cross the water. The land is split in two so they can't go around the lake. Some time the god of the Underworld will use his shape-shifting abilities and will sneak a little hole in the land and will sneak across and destroy it.

The ending is that the Underworld gods are not getting across. Everything is waiting and nothing is changing right now.

# SCAFFOLDING SUPPORT FOR STORYTELLERS

## Support for storytellers in naming mode

Naming-mode stories label setting and characters and hold unstated connections between the players and elements in the sandworld. Stories in this category are missing two components: first, a sense of telos, a trajectory that moves from problem to resolution, and, second, organization by which the story tells how the various components of the world relate to each other. A skill that will scaffold naming-mode storytellers' language development is that of sequencing, a foundational organizational frame which uses temporal order to give the story coherence.

### *Developing skill in sequencing*

Dawson was a six-year-old child with language impairment, evidenced in part by his severe difficulty in sequencing. His storytelling was in an early naming mode, a confused jumble of labels and names. An assessment report from the speech and language pathologist included the recommendation that we teach Dawson the foundational organizational frame of sequencing. A strategy typically suggested for teaching sequencing is to provide the student with ready-made images, which, if ordered correctly, indicate a storyline. Instead of providing Dawson with pictures, I gave him the opportunity to create his own story in the sand, stating in sequence what was developing. His own sandtray images replaced the prepared images of the sequence skills book. For Dawson, working with the images of his own dramatized sandtray play was a far more engaging task than learning to state the sequence of a three-step series of pre-made pictures. In essence, he was being coached in the use of dramatizing mode. After several weeks into the process, a developing awareness of sequencing was evident.

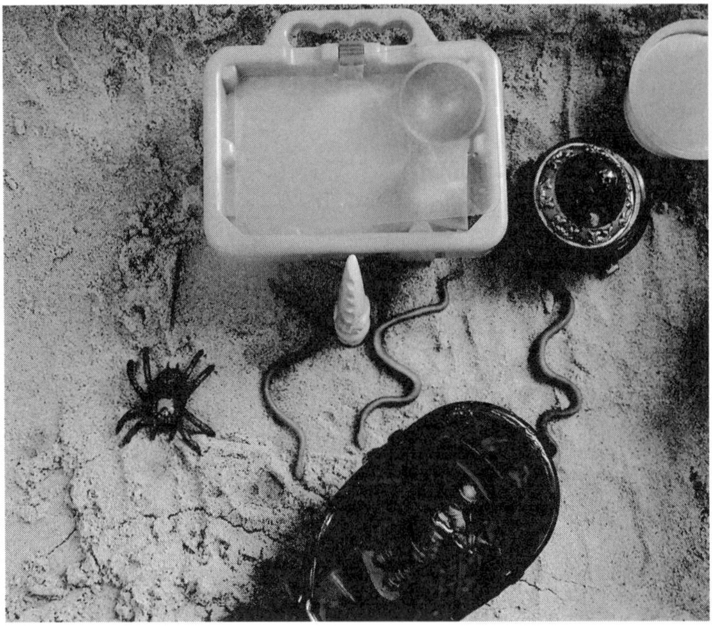

*Figure 4.7 Sandworld at outset of drama*

- Dawson created the world seen in Figure 4.7.
    - 'What is the problem in this world?' the teacher asked, in order to help him give the story an overall coherence by stating the central plot complication.
    - Dawson stated the problem: 'The problem is that the guy needs to try to get through the snakes, the statues, and the spider and kill them so he can have a drink.'
- Dawson dramatized the story while describing the action.
- The teacher wrote down his words, listing the actions as they were spoken, supporting Dawson's sequencing during the telling by supplying the question 'Then what happened?'
- The sandworld scene was modified during the dramatization, eventually becoming the scene pictured in Figure 4.8.

- The teacher then read back the completed story so that Dawson could hear the action as he had sequenced it in his own words.

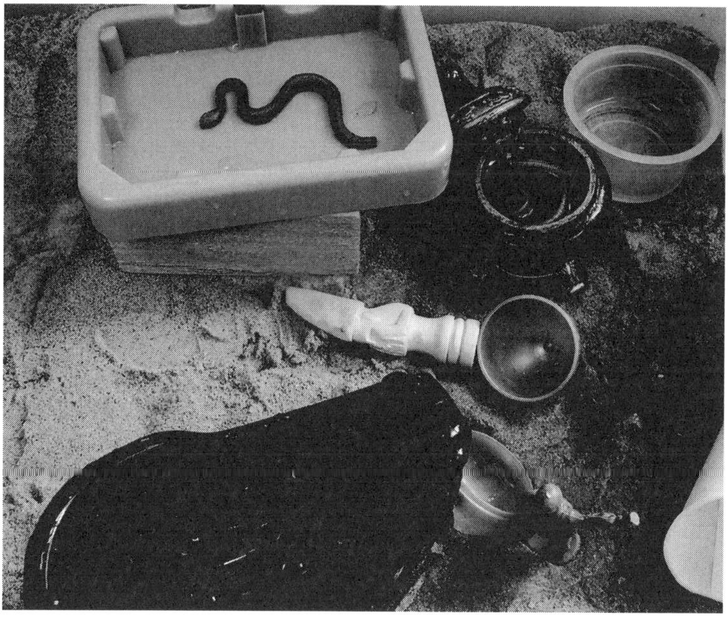

*Figure 4.8 Sandworld after the drama was enacted*

## DAWSON'S STORY

First he moves his ship. Then he jumps out.

He gets the good snake and puts him in the water inside the ship. He puts the bad snakes into the stew pot. Both bad snakes die.

He kills the king statue by hitting him.

He gets to the half eggs. He uses one half to pour the water from the bucket into the egg.

He drinks the water from the egg. He puts the water in the stew so the bad snakes can get hotter and they die.

Dated several weeks into the practice, the story shows that Dawson is beginning to articulate a temporal order as he describes the actions of his story, although, with the repetition of steps three and seven, we can see there was still some confusion – the snakes are boiled twice over! By this time, however, he had made significant gains.

## Support for tellers in dramatizing mode

Life, when we are in the middle of it, is not a story. We 'fly by the seat of our pants', we are 'gobsmacked', we 'play it by ear', we 'muddle our way through', we are 'swept along in the whirlwind', we 'rush headlong into things'. All are kinaesthetic metaphors for experience, which is, by its nature, kinaesthetic. It is later, when we try to talk about it, that the confusion will find a pattern, the embarrassment find humour, the heartache find consolation, the actions find reasons. Only in the telling does the experience become story. Similarly, the story told in dramatizing mode is more experience than narrative as the 'body does the story' and the teller discovers the plot. Like life, the experience that is encountered initially in the blow-by-blow fashion of dramatizing mode can be retold as narrative.

In order to reframe the drama as a narrative, the teller must move beyond the confines of the present tense and articulate connections between characters, events, and emotions. Oral rehearsal in the narrating mode is particularly efficacious in preparing storytellers for writing down the story. Teachers can invite dramatizing-mode storytellers into narrating mode with the following sequence of instructions:

- Today you will think about your story as a movie.
- Choose *one* moment of the movie.
- Freeze-frame it.
- Now tell your story from that moment, the point in time and the place in which the characters are in that one frame.
- Your goal will be *not* to move your hands while telling.
- Let the hearer know the setting and characters.
- Create interest in the listeners so that they want to know how it turns out.

- Make a picture in your mind and grab the listeners' attention.
- Tell it with describing language.
- Tell it in a storyteller's voice.

Told stories enter through the ears. Perhaps the most powerful effect of this exercise is that students hear in their own and in their peers' voices the contrast between two modes of telling.

### *Example of the freeze-frame technique at work*

Ashton has been dramatizing a story in which one scene shows the hero of the story returning home on a raft. He is asked to 'freeze-frame' his story at this point:

> *Teacher:* 'How does the character feel?'
>
> *Ashton:* 'He feels sad but happy because I am going home.'
>
> *Teacher:* 'Well, what did that look like?'
>
> *Ashton:* 'Well, I had a glimmer of hope but he had tears streaming down my face.'
>
> Then Ashton hears what he had just said. His eyes light up: 'OH! So I tell a picture!'

This example is instructive for another reason. The confusion between first- and third-person pronouns shows us that the teller cannot do it all at once. He is learning to work on the word picture to convey the feelings of the character. Next he may address the pronoun issue. I wonder if the pronoun confusion also gives us a glimpse of the storyteller standing in between the inner, undirected and outer, directed thought of the story, the inner thought identifiable by the use of 'I' and 'my' and the directed thought identifiable by the use of 'he'.

## Principles for planning mini-lessons

Over time, storytellers consolidate and expand skills both in structure and in story language. They incorporate the orientation of setting and a problem-solving storyline. They embed character motivation and attributes within the action, begin to use past tense, and start to employ stylistic features such as repetition, rhythm, alliteration, descriptive vocabulary, and dialogue. However, Crystal's 'bucket theory' (1987) argues that a child who is telling a story that is complex at the macrostructural level will trade off some microstructural elements (cited in Justice *et al.* 2006).

### *Choose the focus*

The child cannot do it all at once. As complexity of content goes up, sophistication of articulation goes down and vice versa. A story that has complex plot organization will probably have simple language at the sentence level. Do we want to focus on sentence structure? Episodic organization? Vocabulary usage? We want to focus on all of these, and yet only one at a time. In order to bring a greater richness and fuller satisfaction to the student in expressing what is in imagination, isolate and work with one discrete piece of the setting – one corner of the tray – challenging students to describe how it looks, smells, sounds, feels, or tastes; or one of the three categories of character, problem, or solution, focusing on developing that category; or one character, challenging students to get under the skin or inside the head of that character.

### *Use read-alouds*

Apprentice storytellers are guided and inspired by children's storybook literature. To those who are taught to listen with awareness, the sound of the read-aloud book provides an example of the story cadence, the vocabulary provides a sense of story language, and the plot provides a demonstration of story structure. Dorfman and Capelli (2007) give direction for reading and rereading children's literature to students.

## *Model*

Teacher modeling of the current skill teaching focus is an essential technique. Use of interactive whiteboard technology enables teachers to project the sand pictures of the students to the entire group and model specific storytelling skills. In addition, teacher participation in telling/listening dyads creates opportunity for modeling in the moment as students share their stories orally. In the following example, the teacher responds by labeling with precise vocabulary the objects that are given generic labels in the naming-mode story of a junior kindergarten student.

*Larry:* 'This thing is shooting the ducks.'

*Teacher:* 'I can see the hunter is shooting the ducks.'

*Larry:* 'This guy is driving. This stuff is for the cars to crash into.'

*Teacher:* 'Oh! There's a rampart! And the cars are heading for it!'

*Larry:* 'This thing is moving his legs.'

*Teacher:* 'Is the rhinoceros wiggling his legs?'

Finally, four-year-old Larry states his grand finale: 'All this stuff is going to blow up!'

## *Tie assessment to teaching goal*

Student self and peer checklists create conditions in which collaborative and supportive feedback can flourish. Checklists are tools that reinforce and restate the mini-lesson. Criteria for checklists are couched as restatements of the skills taught in the mini-lesson. A lesson focusing on the ending of the story, for example, might be reinforced with a self-evaluation checklist that states: 'My ending solves the problem in the story. It leaves the listener satisfied.' A lesson focusing on how the teller delivers the story might be accompanied by: 'My partner could hear me. I spoke clearly. I got to the point.'

## *Build awareness that stories are for the teller and stories are for the listener*

There is a subtle but powerful duality here. Stories are told both to express the inner imagination and to communicate in the outer world. Frame your teaching in terms of these two touchstones that address both the teller's experience and how the hearer apprehends the story.

### Stories are for the teller

To the builder's inner eye, the world is layered with colour, with intrigue, danger, sacrifice, pathos, humour, celebration. The articulation of the story may seem abridged and pale in comparison to the richness of the speech and action of the child's imagination. The telling does not as yet do the world justice. This fact informs our teaching; we will try to lead storymakers to a place of satisfaction in communicating to their partners the fullness of their worlds.

Oftentimes the feeling content of the scene is what the sandplayer wants to communicate above all else. The feeling content is the tone of the world, and it may be the underlying or hidden meaning in the scene, the subtext. And because there is not an automatic one-to-one correspondence between feeling and word, finding the right words is particularly gratifying for the teller. One ten-year-old, for example, when telling a dramatized story, repeated like a refrain a single phrase. It captured and communicated a felt sense of foreboding. He spoke the words with evident satisfaction: 'Evil lurking in the shadows.' Here is an excerpt from his story:

---

*Soldier:* This bloodshed does not seem to end. This needless bloodshed and **evil lurking in the shadows**.

*Aside to audience:* The men come across.

*Commander:* Better get back in the tank before danger strikes. Hopefully everything is okay.

*Aside to audience:* This is a war. All this dust and stuff is smoke and stuff.

*Soldier:* Stay! Do not touch the ground! Get away from the tree!

*Men:* We are not enemies; we are friends.

*He moves the soldier, then the horse. Lines up the animals on the right.*

*Soldier:* **There must be evil lurking in the shadows!** I get a bad feeling.

*Men:* We are not the enemy. We will not harm you.

*Soldier:* **The evil lurking in the shadows!** The darkness! The perpetual darkness that has trapped us here on this planet called Earth!

---

### Stories are for the listener

The storyteller needs to step outside her own inner world and imagine how the receiver of the story hears and responds to the telling. Awareness of the listener gives the teller a second perspective from which to form the narrative. Does the beginning pull in the listener? Does the middle keep the listener's attention? Does the ending satisfy the listener? Does the pace of the story mean that the listener does not get bored or frustrated? Is the content appropriate to the listener's stage of development?

I recently listened to a story that captured my interest at the outset. The words were descriptive and were delivered in the cadence of a storyteller. There were interesting characters, conflict, and suspense. But there was a problem with the narrative: every time the story neared the resolution, the teller veered off into another complication. Perhaps she could not find an inner resolution within her own psyche to the problem. 'Stories are for the teller,' I was thinking. But, as listener, I could feel myself holding my breath, inwardly pleading that this time there would be a resolution, and as my impatience increased, I entertained a growing admiration for the peer who seemed to have untiring staying power. This experience formed the basis for a mini-lesson on plot highpoint and resolution, one that was framed from the point of view of 'Stories are for the listener' and was summarized with the slogan 'Get to the point!'

### *Excerpt from a mini-lesson*

It is a little over two weeks into Andrea Slocombe's workshop for a group of Grades 5 (age ten) and 6 (age 11) students. Until this point, the participants have been relying heavily on the labeling and listing of the naming mode. Andrea isolates the beginning section of the story as the focus for the tellers' foray beyond naming into narrating mode.

Over the week prior to this lesson, Andrea has been reading the beginning section of various narratives, giving the students opportunity to hear the sound and analyze the storymaker's technique of engaging the listener at the outset of the story. Andrea reiterates tacitly that stories are for the teller and stories are for the listener. 'Make a picture in your mind' focuses the teller on the inner aspect of storytelling. 'Grab our attention' focuses the teller on the need of the listener who must be reeled in, like a fish, to the alternate world of his narrative. Andrea will follow up this lesson with a student self-evaluation checklist. The checklist reads simply: 'My beginning grabs the listener's attention. It makes him want me to go on.' The use of interactive whiteboard technology enables participants to project their individual storyworlds, providing an opportunity for the entire group to conference together about each story.

> *Andrea:* 'Today you will tell the beginning of your story twice.
>
> First, tell it by labeling what is in your world. Then tell the beginning again, this time with describing language, in a storyteller's voice.
>
> Let the hearers know the setting and characters.
>
> Create interest in the listeners so that they want to hear the rest of the tale.
>
> Make a picture in your mind and grab our attention.'

One by one the sandworlds are projected through the interactive whiteboard as each boy tells the beginning of his story twice – the first time in a naming mode, the second in a narrative mode. The following is the transcript of one boy's contribution.

> *Student:* 'I can't remember everything in my story.'
>
> *Andrea:* 'That's okay.'
>
> *Student:* (*pointing*) 'I'm that guy. I don't have a name for this.'

*Andrea:* 'Walk us through.'

*Student:* 'These are my troops. This is a big Pot of Doom. Here is the enemy side. These are explosives. This is two rockets and a machine gun.'

*Andrea:* 'Now think about the setting and characters. Make a picture in your mind. Grab our attention.'

*Student:* 'I'm good at the writing part but I am having trouble with telling.'

*Andrea:* 'Think about the story!'

*Student:* 'Rocky, dusty, moldy, in the middle of nowhere, just outside the enemy border, we stopped and found the enemy lookout posts. As me and my man, Snipe (he's a sniper), look through to find the enemy, we found a Grab Claw Machine. We wonder if it will ever notice us. Then we see it pick up an MG! We only have one small rocket left. It is just big enough to destroy it.'

*Andrea:* 'Who wants to know what happens next?'

(*Applause, encouraging comments from group.*)

'Here is', 'this is', 'there are', the storyteller begins at first try. Then he begins again, in the new mode. Introducing his story with 'Rocky, dusty, moldy', he engages the hearer imaginatively in the sensory experience of the setting. It works! We feel the choking desert air of his world and its desolation. It is not too much to say that the retelling demonstrates a shift into a richness of vocabulary and the beginnings of suspense, and the language contains hints of a poetic cadence. This storyteller has shifted into a narrating mode. It has happened through the ear: 'Tell it in a storyteller's voice.'

CHAPTER 5

# LISTENING

*'The most important thing about listening is to make sure you understand the story. You have to do that by focusing and asking good questions that help people improve their story. You need to ask the question nicely. Like you wouldn't say, "Where did the forest come from!" You would ask, "Could you explain why the forest is in the story?"'*

– Sandtray Narrative Group (in answer to the end-of-year question: 'What is the most important thing about listening?')

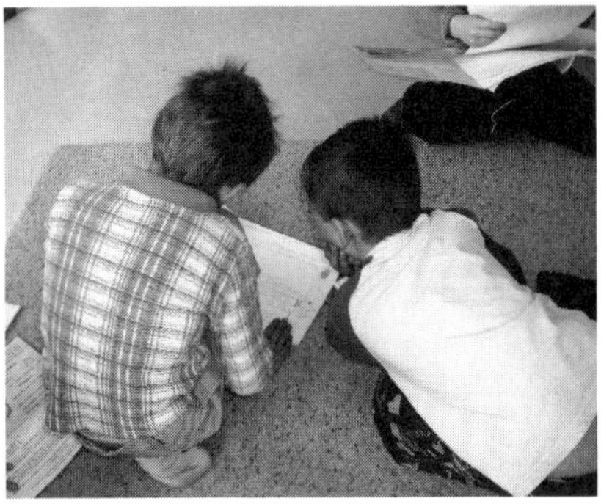

*Figure 5.1a Reading and listening*

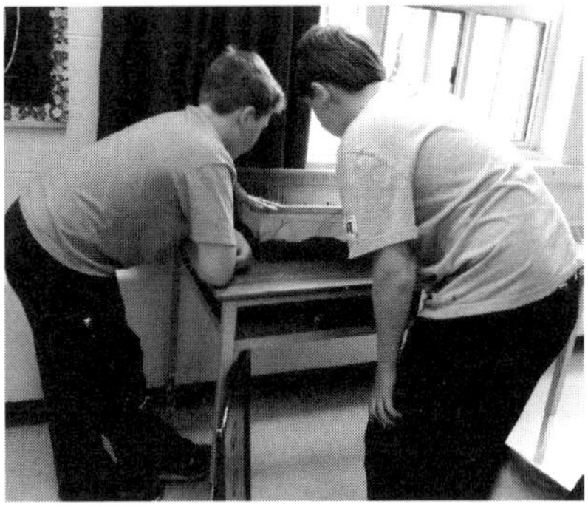

*Figure 5.1b Telling and listening*

'Hunger is kitchen,' my Scottish mother-in-law would say in reply to our thanks after she had served up a bountiful meal. In the same way that a cook needs eager appetites around the supper table, so does a storymaker need a listener. It is hunger for story that invites storymaking.

The master storyteller Joan Bodger reflects on the bond between teller and listener. The listener, she observes, participates in the teller's narrative, and the participation is vital: 'The listener becomes a partner in the creation of another world' (2000, p.266). Story-making and its mirror twin, story-listening, are two sides of one imaginative activity, two sides of the storying coin. There is a reciprocity that is at work between the teller of the tale and the receiver.

This interdependence of telling and listening means that instead of learning how to listen by learning *about* listening, students can learn to listen *by* listening. The skill development happens in real time. The skills of listening are actively taught to students in a sandtray narrative workshop as they practise daily hearing and responding to a peer's story. They receive ongoing training in receptivity.

'Listen to your partner's story' is our instruction to the participant who now is going to hear a partner's narrative, either told or read. 'Then give them two appreciations and ask one question.'

## LISTENING: A WORKSHOP ESSENTIAL

The sandtray workshop is a container, one that enables students to explore unreservedly their individual landscapes, creating a classroom counterpart analogous to the 'free and protected space' (Kalff 1980, p.39) of the sandplay therapy room. Importantly, it is the students themselves who must fashion the environment as a safe place in which worlds can be built and stories can be told and read. The participants must take each other seriously; they need to learn to hear and respond to one another. Mindful partner listening is essential to the workshop's viability. 'We must play,' writes C.S. Lewis, '[b]ut our merriment must be of that kind (and it is, in fact, the merriest kind) which exists between people who have, from the outset, taken each other seriously – no flippancy, no superiority, no presumption' (2005, p.94). The merriment he describes comes with the practice of listening. When the listener begins to say, 'I can put aside my own agenda and take in another's story,' the teller is able to say, 'What I have to say is worthwhile.'

Respectful partner listening and feedback declares to the tellers that they have ideas that matter, an awareness that imbues their experience in class and playground during the entirety of their school day. Participants in one sandtray narrative workshop described the synergy that the telling/listening interrelationship created as the year progressed: 'It became more fun and we got more ideas on things you could do in the sand from our friends when we shared. We became more confident and knew we had good ideas.'

## Importance of listening

The ability to listen not only affects the capacity to relate interpersonally, it also fundamentally impacts potential for academic success.

### *Social/emotional domain*

Because listening is, first of all, a social act, it is implicitly and explicitly connected with the social-emotional development of the child. The ability to listen in a way that receives what the other is saying is essential to social intelligence. Cooperation, empathy, creative problem-solving, and relationship skills require listening competency. Ability to listen results not only in increased skill in attending to and participating within the classroom but also an increased ability to listen to one another on the playground. Estrem (2005) found that preschool boys who were less capable in the area of receptive language were more apt to be physically aggressive (Jalongo 2010, p.6). The child in the playground who has learned to listen with attention is equipped with a primary tool in collaborative conflict resolution (Bodine and Crawford 1998).

### *Academic domain*

Mary Renck Jalongo's helpful synthesis of recent literature in the field of listening in early childhood (2010) cites research by Cruger (2005) that demonstrates that children's ability to comprehend what they hear is highly predictive of academic achievement and, conversely, that children with poor auditory comprehension are at risk for failure, more likely to fall behind their peers as the years go by and academic demands increase. The net result of poor receptive language is poor behaviour spawned by disengagement, and the net result of good receptive language is engaged behaviour energized by involvement in the aural life of the classroom (pp.4–6). It is not surprising that the child who cannot keep up with the pace and content of group discussion or follow the teacher's verbal instructions will be at risk academically. Any one of us doomed to listen to input that we do not understand will become bored and either withdraw into our own worlds or find ways to entertain ourselves. Conversely, when we listen with comprehension, we are engaged and able to participate. The capacity to listen determines an upward or downward spiral in our learning.

## What is listening?

Hearing becomes an act of listening when we give attention to what we hear. Clark (2005) defines listening as 'a form of communication that involves hearing, interpreting, and constructing meanings: an active process that is not limited to the spoken word; and an essential way of participating in daily routines as well as in wider decision-making processes' (Jalongo 2010, p.2). Listening is a far-reaching skill that involves not only receiving auditory input but also making meaning of what is heard. It is not passive but active.[1] Listening demands intention. The actions of listening might be characterized as:

- setting aside an impulse to formulate a response while another is speaking
- assuming that the other may have something to say that is not already in our purview
- being open to meeting a different reality from the preconceived one.

Take, for example, the biblical story of Samuel. In the story, a boy is roused from sleep with the sound of a voice calling his name. Each time the boy assumes it is his teacher. He goes to his teacher, Eli, and

1 Thomas Gordon in his book *Leader Effectiveness Training* (1977) coined the term 'Active Listening', a designation that refers to Gordon's suggestion that the listener 'need only restate, in their own language, their impression of the expression of the sender' (p.57). Here I am not referring to the technique taught by Gordon, and expanded in the practice of Nonviolent Communication (Rosenberg 1999) as 'receiving empathetically' (p.78). Rather, I merely wish to distinguish between hearing as passive reception and listening as intentional.

asks what he needs. After the third visit from the boy, Eli instructs Samuel that the next time he is awakened, he should reply, 'Speak, Lord, for your servant is listening' (1 Samuel 3:9). The teacher is instructing the boy in the act of listening as a stance of openness, awareness, discrimination, and perception.

## ONE MORNING: A CIRCLE OF LISTENING

Five six- and seven-year-old students, re-entering the routine of school after a long, hot holiday weekend, sit on the floor in a tight circle.

Eva begins the conversation. Her family went last night to say goodbye to an uncle and aunt who are, she said, 'splitting up' after seven years. 'We went to wish them a good life,' she says.

David shakes his head, over and over. 'That is really sad. That is really, really sad.' The children sit in silent agreement. Over in the corner, the whirring of the fan becomes a distinct tick, tick, tick. After a while, David has something to say. Last weekend he went into the forest and found a ball. A round ball. He shows the roundness with his hands. His brand new teeth are jagged. He has a jack o'lantern mouth and luminous eyes.

'What colour was the ball?' someone asks.

'Gold! It was gold!' He pauses. 'And you open it up.' He shows with his hands the ball opening up. 'And there's a little round thing inside it. Like a treasure.'

'What did you do with it?'

'I buried it back again, by a little pond. I know where it is so I can dig it up again.'

Connie speaks next. 'I know what! I think we should just talk about sad things today.' She looks around the circle: 'My grandma died this past winter. She had cancer. It was gone, we thought. We thought she was getting better, but then she went to the hospital. She died all by herself in her bed in the hospital. Then they buried her.' She pauses. 'I don't know what happens when they bury you.'

Again the children sit in deep sympathy and wordless comfort. Harriet says she has a 'connection' to what Connie said. 'My grandpa's body just got worn out. Old. And so he just passed out on the floor. Just like that. He died.' She shrugs as if to say, 'That is that.'

Karl, who had been waiting, now finds the words: 'This winter I went on a trip to where my real mom lives. I went to see her again. But she got in an accident and she died. And I didn't see her. And the same with Auntie, she died.'

Moments pass. At the window the breeze bumps the Venetian blinds against the sill. The school band down the hall sounds faint and far away. Eventually David responds, 'Oh, that is a bad thing. Really bad.'

I get a small bottle of lotion.[2] 'Karl, I'm glad you are here. Any hurts today?' He points to a little scratch on his finger. I give a dab of lotion for him to apply to his scratch. 'Hurrah for Karl!' we all say, and I touch hands with him in a gentle high five. In turn, Karl repeats the words and actions with Eva, who sits beside him. The ritual of consolation continues, child to child, around the circle.

The circle disperses.

I know that the children have named mysteries this morning. More than that, they have listened to each other. Listening, given child to child, actively and intently, without judgment or the need to assign a solution – that has been their gift to each other.

Although listening is foundational for both academic and social success, and although it is the language skill first learned and most used, it is often not taught explicitly within the school system. We hear in our classrooms the teacher's instruction to 'listen carefully', but little accompanying instruction on how to do so. Perhaps because listening is ubiquitous, because it happens anyway, because it is invisible, and because it is difficult to assess, we have relegated it to the position of the poor cousin of reading, writing, and speaking in our classrooms.

Like the teacher in the story of Samuel, we must help our students learn to listen. This is not an easy task. Children of this century have the sensory input for entertainment and distraction and communication attached to their ears and lying in the palms of their hands. Fallow

2 An adaptation of the group Theraplay entry ritual of 'Checkups' described in Rubin (2001, p.371).

moments may be rarities. Ironically, all this hearing may train our children not to listen. How do we teach this discriminating, responsive act in a society when silence is rare, when hearing is passive? How do we teach our children, in Rumi's words, to 'bring the talky business to an end' (1995, p.198)? We teach them to listen when we give them something that engages their heart and grips their imagination: we give them stories.

## STRATEGIES TO SUPPORT LISTENING LEARNING

### Instructions for listeners in the workshop

- Listen to your partner's story (see listening guidelines below: eyes, ears, mouth, whole body, hands, head).
- After you have heard the story, ask yourself: What are two things that really stood out for me, that I really liked about this story? These are your appreciations.
- Then think: What is it that I want to know more about, that I am not understanding? What am I confused about? This is your question.
- Give your partner two appreciations and one question.
- Exchange roles. Move to the sandtray of the partner who was the listener and exchange roles.
- If you are conferring about a written story, the format of sharing and response is the same: two appreciations, one question, and exchange roles.

#### *A closer look at two appreciations and one question*

The structure of the workshop ensures that the students learn the discipline of noticing the positive aspects of peers' work and learn the skill of translating critique into question.

- *Two appreciations:* To offer two appreciations, listeners must understand, interpret, and evaluate the details of the partner's world and the story. Only someone who has been listening can do this. The term 'appreciation' carries the presumption of gratitude. In my mind, appreciation is preferable to the term 'praise', which may have the nuance of superiority; the giver of praise is assumed to be in a position to judge and determine what is praiseworthy. The ratio of two observations to one question, as well as the order of appreciation before question, ensures that the listener approaches the teller with receptivity. This works against the impulse of the listener to jump in with a critical mindset immediately upon hearing a story.

- *One question:* The question gives weight and importance to the telling. The motive of the questioner is not to give a veiled suggestion to the teller, but to gain increased understanding. The question seeks clarification, confirmation, or information. Sometimes an apparent contradiction in the story needs to be explicated. Setting, characters, relationship between characters, motivations, problem, resolution, the climax of the plot – any of these areas may be addressed by the listener who may want to have more information or further description.

## Reference physical cues

Listening is an activity of the whole body. Eyes, ears, mouth are all engaged. It is important, then, to teach listening by engaging the awareness of the whole body. Display a poster with the following guidelines and expand the students' understanding using the physical cues as suggested below.

LISTENING GUIDELINES

- **Eyes** Look at the speaker and their sandworld
- **Ears** Listen
- **Mouth** Do not interrupt
- **Whole body** Give attention with your whole self
- **Hands** Keep your hands out of the speaker's world
- **Head** Think: What do you appreciate? What do you want clarified?

An elaboration of the poster might include an explanation such as follows:

- *Eyes:* Look at the speaker and his world. Your eyes do not roam around the room. Remember how it feels on the schoolyard if the person you are talking to is scanning the territory around or beyond you. You feel that person is thinking about someone or something other than you.
- *Ears:* It is the time for putting your own story into the corner of your mind and opening your ears to your partner's story. It means that you jump on your partner's story train and ride it. Find out where the story is taking you. Give way. Get into the groove. Let your ears take it all in.
- *Mouth:* Do not interrupt with your own words. Put your opinions on hold. It is not the time for speaking. Let your partner finish the tale before you speak. You must not intrude into your partner's world or story. It is her story, her world. She is the one with the power to name the good and the bad, the hope and the fear, the problem and the resolution, the love and the hate. She is telling her story. You are privileged to listen and to wait.
- *Whole body:* Give attention with your whole self. The storymaker needs to know that you are really hearing him, really seeing his world and really feeling the problems and hopes and fears of its citizens. The storymaker will know all of this when you let your body just lean forward and get into the moment.
- *Hands:* Keep your hands out of your partner's world. It is not your domain. It is not yours to enter; it is yours to observe and appreciate. It is under the governorship of the storyteller. You are an invited guest. You have a passport, and that is your imagination. You are walking the forests and hills of another's world. You treat it with respect.
- *Head:* Get into your partner's world in your imagination. How does it feel? What do you wish could happen? What is

surprising you? What is delighting you? What do you make a connection with? What do you not understand? What feels confusing? What is it that you want to know more about in this world?

## Role play

In the mini-lesson, create dramatizations of listening situations. Role-play bad listening behaviours while a student volunteer relates an anecdote to you. Demonstrate the gamut of poor listening body language (looking around, interrupting, extraneous questions, interrupting, fidgeting, waving at someone across the room). Next, follow the demonstration of poor listening with a demonstration of focused listening (eyes, ears, leaning forward in an interested posture). Make sure that it is you, the teacher, who impersonates the poor listener, not the student. Ask speaker and audience for emotional reactions after each role play. Both audience and participants will experience viscerally the contrast between the two attitudes of listening.

## Narrow the focus

A narrative has a structure comprising of an orientation that sets the scene by introducing characters and setting, a complication or problem that builds and is told through a sequence of action and the interaction of the characters in the story, and, finally, a resolution that satisfies. From time to time, instruct students to direct their feedback to one segment of the story: characters, setting, problem, or solution. Questions can help the teller to unearth the unstated background story of the character, can help him focus on one part of the setting, take time to articulate what the problem might hold, build satisfaction in the resolution, or 'zoom in' on one 'Small Moment' (Calkins and Oxenhorn 2003, p.12). Raise awareness of question words by connecting them to their possible territories:

Who? ______________________________ (Characters)

What? Why?________________________ (Problem)

Where? When? ____________________ (Setting)

How? __________________________ (Solution)

## Model and coach

Model the 'two appreciations, one question' response format. Make students aware of the difference between flaccid and non-specific words, such as 'nice', and words that communicate with nuance. Model the difference between open-ended and closed questions. Computer technology can expand the format in which we can listen to stories and give feedback. Interactive whiteboard technology opens up a world of possibility for mini-lessons. With the sandtrays projected on screen, an entire group of students can listen and give focused feedback to the teller, supported by teacher modeling and feedback in the moment. Online discussion tools that focus on media provide opportunities for users to upload pictures of their sandworlds and record their stories. Listeners to the story can share feedback, using voice with a microphone or telephone, text, audio file, or video via a webcam. Students post their sandworld stories online and receive peer and teacher feedback.

## Example of a listener's question evoking rich language in Grade 6 (age 11)

Appreciations and questions can help a teller who is telling in the naming mode (see Chapter 4) to unfold the unstated meaning behind the label. In the following example, simple questioning elicits a satisfying portrayal of the characters and setting. The teller moves from a flat, one-dimensional listing of elements in her story to a vibrant description of a world teaming with activity, exuberance, and danger.

The story begins with a list:

- giant
- witch

- spider
- pixie
- market.

*Questioner:* 'What are they like?'

*Response:* 'Giants can be good. When they get angry they start throwing stuff. They don't understand.

The witch is tiny because she is the only human. Seen from another planet (where we are), she is very tiny. She feels happy because she is magical. She turns people into frogs. She can make herself grow as tall as a tower. Makes a brew into a pot that is alive. The soup can be the veins inside the pot. That is a good thing for a spider bite because then the poison is not effective.

The spiders are vicious, poisonous. They will bite you if you come too close.

A pixie can be mean.

A market is where you buy anything. The market is also beside the sign that says "Danger". At the market, you can buy fairies, food, toys, diamonds, emeralds, erasers, pencils, clothing, sand, rocks, pixies, spiders. You can even buy people.

For *money* you can use sandstones, sand tablets. You get the sandstone money in The Unknown. There falls from the sky in The Unknown, gold mines, cows, children, sandstones. It is like: "I'M RICH!"'

### *Example of listener question to clarify plot in junior kindergarten*

Holden, Jess, and Ned are sharing their stories.

*Holden:* 'This is sinking sand. This is T-Rex. This is something that is for rocks.'

*Teacher:* 'A catapult.'

*Holden:* 'Yes, a catapult.'

Ned wants to ask a question. Teacher reminds him of the question words: who, what, where, when, why, or how.

*Ned:* 'How did those guys get in the sinking sand?'

*Holden:* 'Because they did not know it was sinking sand. They went in there and they did not understand what it was.'

## Time frame

- After building their sandworlds, which takes approximately 15 to 25 minutes, give the students the signal to move into their telling/listening dyads.
- Facilitate the builder's transition to the phase of telling and listening with a five-minute warning. There may be no need for a whole-group announcement terminating the building section, but a gentle and individual reminder to 'wrap up' in five minutes.
- Provide a cue with a *visual clock* or draw a clock that shows the end time so that the student sees the parameters in which he has to work.
- At the site of the sandtray, the builder tells the story of the sandworld to the partner who listens and then responds with two positive comments and one question.
- If the workshop incorporates writing as well as telling into its format, there will be two arenas for the activity of listening: peer conferencing in response to the told story and in response to the written story. Two possible time structures are offered below. The first is a time frame of 45 minutes that incorporates the telling/listening only. The second is a time frame of 90 minutes that incorporates the written component and has, therefore, two listening segments embedded within it (Figure 5.2). Both structures suggest a mid-workshop gathering for the mini-lesson. However, every class is different, and teachers develop time structures that meet the needs of individual groups. Not every group needs a mini-lesson every day.

45-MINUTE WORKSHOP WITH
TELLING/LISTENING ONLY

*Greeting:* 5 minutes
*Building:* 15–25 minutes
*Reciprocal sharing (telling and listening):* 10–15 minutes
*Gathering* for mini-lesson (optional): 5–10 minutes
*Cleanup and farewell:* 5–10 minutes

90-MINUTE WORKSHOP WITH TELLING
AND RECORDING

*Greeting:* 5 minutes
*Building:* 20–25 minutes
*Reciprocal sharing (telling and listening):* 10–15 minutes
*Gathering* for mini-lesson: 10–15 minutes
*Writing and peer conferencing:* 30 minutes
*Cleanup and farewell:* 5–10 minutes
*Adjust time allotment according to student age and needs.

*Figure 5.2 Two possible time frames – 45 minutes and 90 minutes*

### *Listening to the written story*

A workshop that incorporates a writing segment includes peer conferencing in response to the writer's readiness for the feedback from a peer. It happens in response to writer request. It may not, therefore, happen on a daily basis. Students confer with partners at times when particular stories have reached a phase that requires feedback for revision. This means that the class does not move as a single body through the activities of the workshop. Rather, the flow of events is determined by the needs of the individuals. Students place their name on a list to indicate that they want a peer conference and meet when a peer becomes available.

## Assessment of listening

Because assessment is continuously woven into both teaching and learning in a cycle in which assessment of student learning informs our next steps in teaching, assessment is tied to the current mini-lesson topic. Assessment 'look-fors' are constantly evolving to reflect current teaching and learning goals.

The specific skill that the teacher assesses in observations, anecdotal records, and checklists is the skill the children themselves are stepping back to evaluate in their self- and peer-evaluation checklists. This coordination of teacher and student focus ensures that the students are involved in their own learning, that they are part of the process, that assessment is a tool that clarifies how they can improve.

- The checklist focuses the workshop participants on the specific components of the skill taught in the current mini-lesson, thereby reinforcing what is addressed in the mini-lesson.
- By providing the checklist, teachers are transparent in telling the students what they are working on.
- Self- and peer-evaluation direct student attention to success criteria. Students apply and assimilate what they have heard.
- Checklists not only invite awareness of the component skills of listening but also bring users to the next step of strategic use.
- Checklists develop accountability and foster metacognitive awareness.
- Note that the peer-evaluation checklist example in Figure 5.3 uses a gradient of stars and a 'Not yet' category. The use of stars delimits the evaluation to a positive critique. The checklist category of 'Not yet' reinforces the tacit assumption that the learning will take place. This frame supports a classroom ethos, described by Jones as one in which 'children can take risks without fear of reprisals and where a spirit of mutual respect and exploration is valued' (2007, p.572).

| My partner… | ★★ | ★ | Not yet |
|---|---|---|---|
| Kept eyes on me and my world | | | |
| Nodded and showed listening with body language | | | |
| Gave two appreciations that made sense to me | | | |
| Asked me a question that helped me think further about my story | | | |

*Figure 5.3 Sample peer evaluation listening checklist used in Andrea Slocombe's workshop*

## THE FRUITS OF LISTENING LEARNING: EXAMPLES FROM THE SPECIAL EDUCATION RESOURCE ROOM

The classroom that fosters skills in listening will make possible surprising moments of meeting between its members. A collaboration that successfully spanned the divide between Grade 7 and Kindergarten, a dialogue between seven-year-olds akin to what we might expect of a writer's salon, and the offering of support in place of antipathy – all are examples of such meetings. The meetings are chronicled below. In each situation the students had been trained to listen to each other.

## Building communication across grades

I invited an intermediate-age student struggling with school phobia to be a peer helper (Figure 5.4) in a workshop comprising of five junior kindergarten students, some of whom were identified with expressive language difficulties, one of whom displayed selective mutism, one of whom was struggling with behavioural challenges.

The experiment worked largely because of the lack of condescension in the attitude of the older student towards the younger ones in her intentional listening and feedback to the stories of their sandworlds. In the following exchange, her respect towards the drama of the kindergartener's world and the seriousness with which she asks her questions are evident.

> *JK student:* 'Er' amamals in there. Er' ant in there. Ant is going over to bite Mickey Mouse. Er' dolphin is swimming. Coming over.'
>
> *Peer helper:* 'I really like how you set up this.' (*Points to figurine of lady with dinosaur figurine placed facing her in a threatening position.*)
>
> *JK student:* 'The dolphin is comes over.' (*She moves the dolphin and puts it on top of the dinosaur's head.*)
>
> *Teacher:* 'The dolphin is coming over to protect the lady.'
>
> *Peer helper: 'Do you think the dinosaur could be saving Mickey Mouse?'*
>
> *JK:* 'NO! NO! The *dolphin* is saving Mickey Mouse.'

The peer helper now tells her own story to two of the kindergarten children. An excerpt of it is below. What is noteworthy in the exchange is the listening response of the kindergarten student. The four-year-old child's response – 'The princess is trapped in her cave grave' – is a masterful paraphrase of the central problem of the story and the feeling content it contains. The older student feels that her story is heard and understood.

> *Peer helper:* (*pointing*) 'Here there is not a specific door you are supposed to go in and there is no way out of it.'
>
> *JK student:* 'The princess is trapped in her cave grave?'
>
> *Peer helper:* 'YES!'

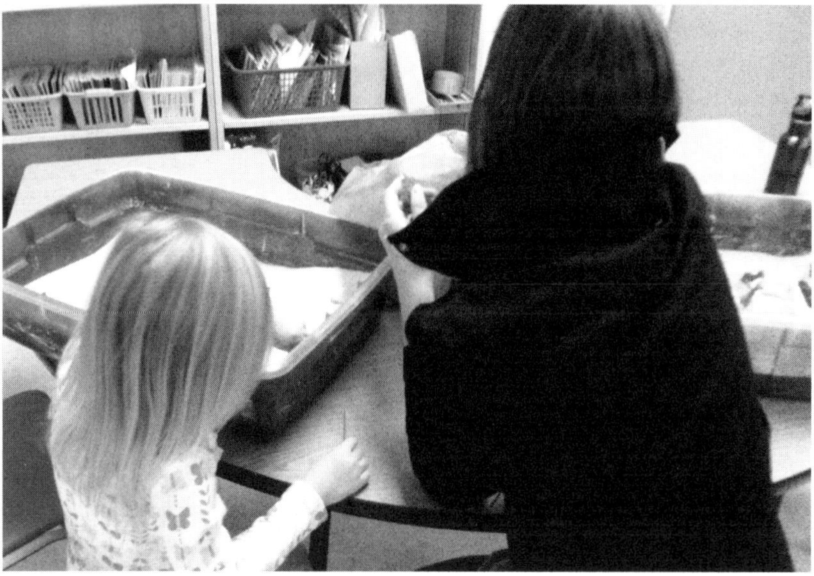

*Figure 5.4 Building listening communication in junior kindergarten/Grade 7 (age 12) dyad*

## Fostering a writers' dialogue

The listening classroom fosters a dialogue in which one writer's voice speaks in response to another. The following incident took place on Earth Day. That day Munan did not write a narrative. Instead, he wrote about the beauty and fragility of the earth in a piece reminiscent of an environmentalist's instructional manual.

THE EARTH

The earth is Big and round too. The rain falls on this beautiful planet. Maybe you can save the Earth because people are littering on this beautiful planet. This make Mother Earth feel sick. The look is not good for outer space. The Earth is small planet but the Earth too is big because we are small and our school had a clean up and all of our town. Everybody on Earth is cleaning even me and I love it because the Earth is clean. The Earth has many colours.

When Munan shared this piece of writing in a mid-workshop group sharing time, the Grade 2 (age seven) students listened intently. Myles, in particular, was moved by this piece. Like a participant in a writers' salon, he returned to his desk and wrote, 'I have a litil pom myself' (Figure 5.5). His response to Munan's writing expresses a contentment mixed with wonder that all is well, that he has a best friend, that he lives in beauty.

---

ERTH DAY

My firand Munan made me feel very happey about erth day. I have a litil pom myself. I am so lucey to have this world. it is budiful. me and Munan are best friends. the world is budiful.

---

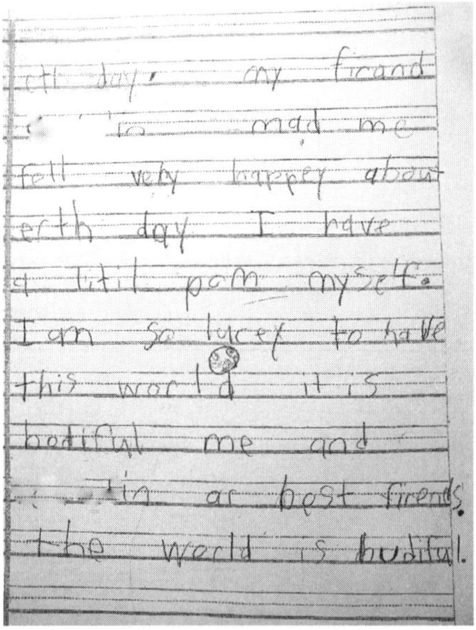
erth day. my firand
mad me
fell very happey about
erth day I have
a litil pom myself.
I am so lucey to have
this world it is
bodiful me and
ar best firends.
the world is budiful.

*Figure 5.5 'I have a litil pom myself'*

## Replacing patterns of rejection with patterns of support

Veterans of social skills groups may be highly skilled at talking about feelings and understanding conflict resolution scenarios, skillful with the lingo of non-violent communication, insightful about their own behaviours. Many have learned a second language of empathy and assertiveness, much as they would memorize verbs in French or Spanish language class. In fact, they may have become fluent.

But learning a new language is not enough. More needs to transpire in the group than rehearsal of appropriate interactions and language. My sense is that skill groups are effective – transformative, even – when there is an experience of deep acceptance, when the group facilitates an encounter rather than merely a rehearsal, when the group is a safe place as much as a teaching place, when there is a lived experience of giving empathy rather than merely talking about empathy.

This experience is what was offered to one small group of six- and seven-year-old girls who had fallen prey to intense rivalry and in-fighting and were locked in a pattern of rotating victimization that blamed first one student, then another. They participated in a small-group, weekly session of sandtray play that included a group welcoming circle, individual building, telling, listening, and responding in the group of four. From time to time, the girls produced a written record of their told stories.

An early story written by each member of the group is included below. Respectively, the stories chronicle helplessness, the fruitless search for a key, blaming, and punishment.

---

*Student 1:* There was a planet called the Planet of Narnea. It had a dinosaur and his name was Odney because he always gets hurt. even today. and three cats wear driving and got stuck in singking Sand. The balurena was dancing and fell into the singking sand. So she died. The End.

*Student 2:* Once there was key to press a bottom in the Dinasors house. It was a shell key but the anemals cudent find the key. thay looked and looked but thay culd not find it at all. so the snake tried to find it but stons falled on him and he Died. The End.

*Student 3:* It is November! The dog blamd it on the hourse. But the dog he did it. the dog hided the treshor.

*Student 4:* Once upon a time there was 2 dogs, cat's, two zebras, house, polar bier, clocks, shel's, beds. All animals are sleeping. The cat is garding in the night. If they are hungry and wake up the queen zaps the animals. A bell rings when thay wake up.

In the initial three minutes of the first group meeting, the participants were quarrelling. The topic at hand was their sitting posture. They were disagreeing about who was the initiator, who was the imitator: *I thought of it first... No, I did... Did not... I did.*

In order to practise listening receptivity, each session was designed to begin with an adaptation of the ritual of 'Checkups' described in Phyllis Rubin's chapter entitled 'Group Theraplay' (in Jernberg and Booth) in which each child has 'a "moment in the spotlight" when she is recognized, admired, and cared for without having to ask for it' (2001, p.371). We sat in a circle and each girl, in turn, greeted and responded to the person beside her.

'Hello, Stacey,' I might begin. 'Glad you are here. Any hurts today?'

'No!' Stacey might reply.

The entire group would respond: 'No hurts! Hurrah! High five!'

The first girl (let's call her Jasmine) would then give Stacey a high five.

Alternatively, Stacey's reply might be 'Yes!' and she might point out a visible or invisible hurt (located between fingers and elbows, toes and knees). In response to this, Jasmine would give her a dab of lotion to apply around the designated spot. After her lotion application, the group would declare 'Hurrah for Stacey! High five!'

Stacey, the recipient of attention, now would turn to the one beside her, continuing the pattern with the same greeting: 'Hello, Manuela, glad you're here. Any hurts today?'

This ritual would continue around the circle, until each member had been both giver and recipient of the caring question: 'Hello! Any hurts? Hurrah! High five!'

This was nurturing listening, given simply and eloquently, student to student, with few words. It was a powerful corrective to the habit of rivalry.

Following the opening ritual, the 'build, tell, listen, and respond' sequence defined the format of the workshop. Because these particular students were so accustomed to criticizing each other, it was crucial that there be teacher presence during the listening and responding.

In order to enable teacher modeling and monitoring of supportive responses and questions, the listening segment took place not with one partner but with the entire group of four. The listening task was challenging because it was necessary for these students to relinquish the reflexive put-downs, to enter imaginatively into another's world, and to reflect on it in order to respond with positive feedback and interested questions.

Not only was listening a challenge but so also was building and telling. Building a world was outside the comfort zone of these children because the required solitude derailed their habit of comparing their own work with their peers' productions while in process. Telling the story took courage because the moment of revealing the story world was the moment of vulnerability. Sharing it required trusting the group's receptivity. However, in spite of the challenging nature of the process, the girls were intrigued and invigorated by it.

The transformative work with this small group took place because their listening was not a rehearsal. In a few months, by practising receptive listening both in opening circle and in story sharing, the girls began to see one another as vulnerable, and as allies, not competitors. In time, they became a friendship group that sustained a supportive attitude in class, an attitude that eventually they carried with them into the playground.

Chapter 6

# WRITING

*'We get really into the story and want to share it with family and friends, then we want to write it down.'*

– Grade 5 (age ten) and 6 (age 11) workshop students (in answer to the end-of-year question: 'What was the most important thing about recording the story?')

Building a world, telling the story it contains, hearing and responding to another's story – together these segments comprise a workshop, complete and entire.

But storymakers have an innate impulse to preserve their stories. A workshop that devotes time to writing will answer the maker's desire, harness the energy of story, and take advantage of an inestimable opportunity for teaching the craft of writing.

## CHALLENGES TO WRITING

'Writing? I HATE writing!' Carla blurts out. This is the first day of sandtray storymaking and she has just heard the overview of what will be expected. A captive receiving the sentence of 20 years' hard labour might have responded in the same heartfelt tones. The sidelong looks of the other children and their furtive smiles tell me that she has voiced a common sentiment, so I do not refer again to writing the story after telling it, but to preserving a record. I call it 'recording'.

The fact is that all too often when we assign a written language activity, eyes like Carla's glaze over, energy drains away, efforts are desultory. We find students sitting in front of paper or computer, staring at a blank field. Writing tasks trigger predictably defiant responses in children who display oppositional behaviour, making it commonplace knowledge among teachers that there is a correlation between behaviour flare-ups and writing difficulties. Teachers interviewed in one school painted a picture of their frustration in the comments below:

> He usually just sits in writing class and stares at the ceiling or plays with something in his hands... He doesn't write, he runs... Refuses to turn on her computer... If she writes, it is so short and minimal it is difficult to mark... Engages in the literacy block, but when the writing portion comes along he will get anxious, blow up or walk out... She refuses to write and also refuses to have people scribe for her... If you try to address his work refusal, it will turn into a huge battle... He will not write at all in class. Only scribing.

Writing demands discrete skills, as students must become adept both at using a given knowledge base – spelling rules and punctuation, for example – and at organizing the content of their thoughts. For children, frustration with inability to access ideas, shame at what they perceive as an inferior appearance of the end product, or a physical struggle with small-motor tasks may spawn reluctance to approach the tasks of written language. Language learning disabilities, fine-motor disorders, self-definition, habits of mind, a history of failure, a history of teachers choosing to focus on the mechanics of spelling and punctuation instead of on the content – all may impact the writer.

Reluctant writers at mid-elementary school level, interviewed at the outset of a sandtray narrative workshop series, describe their experience with writing:

> My words aren't good but I have good ideas... I just can't get my ideas out... I'd rather do stuff than sit and read and write... I don't like anything I am doing... I'm not the hardest worker when I really don't want to do it... I can't write neatly but I know I have good ideas.

Interviewed prior to the sandplay narrative workshop, the students report on frustration, discouragement, and withdrawal. At end-of-year, the same students reflect on what they gleaned over several months of recording sandworld stories. There has been a sea change. We see that the recording of stories that have emerged out of the sandtray is a task that is invested with energy, the energy of the stories themselves. Even the most reluctant want to write down the stories that are their own.

## WRITING IN THE SAND/STORY WORKSHOP: STUDENTS' END-OF-YEAR OBSERVATIONS

### WHAT WAS THE MOST IMPORTANT THING FOR YOU ABOUT RECORDING THE STORY?

- We get really into the story and want to share it with family and friends, then we want to write it down.
- The most important thing about recording is the chance to keep memories of the building that you did.
- Writing helps you become a better teller.
- You can edit your writing to make it sound better than your telling.
- Building is fun and helps people be creative. It helps with your writing because you have the story in your mind while you are building so you don't have to create the story when you are writing.

### WHAT WAS THE BIGGEST HELP IN LEARNING TO RECORD YOUR STORIES?

- Learning that it was important just to get ideas out and not worry about waiting for the best idea helped get the recording started.
- Knowing not to worry about spelling or having the best vocabulary from the very beginning helped us get going.
- Knowing we can go back and bump up our writing, edit with each other, and take out or improve our ideas helped us record our stories and not get stuck.
- Basically, learning that all our ideas are important and it is okay to let them all fly out. It doesn't always have to be the best idea first.

IF YOU WERE DESIGNING A WORKSHOP, WHAT WOULD YOU KEEP THE SAME? WHAT WOULD YOU CHANGE?

- What we would keep the same: Keep the arrangement of the classroom the same. The music should stay the same. Keep doing different ways of recording like animations.
- What we would change: Add more time to write! Make the time in workshop longer because we get into the story and then you have to log off.

## DESIRE, PROCESS, AND FREEDOM: A SANDTRAY NARRATIVE GROUP GUIDES OUR REFLECTIONS ABOUT WRITING

Taking a closer look at the students' end-of-year comments, we find some essentials to consider when bringing students to the phase of writing the story – the role of desire, the place of writing within the larger workshop process, and the prerequisite for freedom from anxiety.

### The role of desire

The energy of desire fuels the writing process:

- *The desire to keep and to communicate:* 'The most important thing about recording is the chance to keep memories of the building that you did.'

  The desire to preserve experience in memory is akin to the journaling impulse to record and document. The story is something these students have experienced viscerally (*we really get into the story*) and they yearn to communicate it with people who are meaningful to them (*and want to share it with family and friends*). The energy to share comes out of the wellspring of connectedness both to the story and to the audience.

- *The desire for a full record:* 'It is important to stay focused and not to rush, so that you include all the details from your telling.'

  In the observation that 'it is important to stay focused and not to rush', the students allude to barriers all too familiar to them including a difficulty with focus, with memory, and with sustaining attention. The abilities to focus, to sustain attention, and to remember are all required in order to master the various skills of phonological awareness, the encoding of sounds with memorized visual symbols, the sequencing of words in a sentence, and remembering the story details.

Vygotsky elucidates the challenge:

> Writing...requires deliberate analytic action on the part of the child. In speaking he is hardly conscious of the sounds he pronounces and quite unconscious of the mental operations he performs. In writing he must take cognizance of the sound structure of each word, dissect it, and reproduce it in alphabetical symbols, which he must have studied and memorized before. In the same deliberate way, he must put words in a certain sequence to form a sentence. (1934/1986, p.182)

Requiring, as it does, such a wide-ranging set of skills, the task of recording the story is large and especially difficult for students who struggle with any of the prerequisite capabilities. When they tell us earnestly that the spoken words of the story (*all the details of the telling*) must be encoded into print or they will be lost, they are saying that it is the feeling of pride in the told narrative, devotion to the story itself, that energizes their efforts in the face of the challenges.

## The creative process

There is a seamless interrelatedness in the cycle of build, tell, and record.

- *Impact of building on writing:* 'Building...helps with your writing because you have the story in your mind while you are building so you don't have to create the story when you are writing.'

As described by the students in this comment, making story is a two-step process – step 1: form ideas while building; step 2: record. The process of discovery of ideas through action is key because students who struggle with various facets of written language are hard-pressed to discover their ideas through writing. The action itself is too onerous a task, and energy is poured into the translating of phonemes into graphemes among other tasks. As Krashen observes, 'Writers who have not mastered the composing process have a much harder time coming up with new ideas' (2003, p.76). They can, however, experience ideas by means of building. Ideas are sparked as the sandworld is created. Writing the story publishes ideas that have been engendered through play and developed through telling.

- *Impact of writing on storytelling:* 'Writing helps you become a better teller.'

  At first blush, this may seem a surprising observation. Gordon Wells offers a comment that is perhaps illuminative of their observation when he notes that 'writing is, par excellence, the activity in which we consciously wrestle with thoughts and words in order to discover what we mean' (1986, p.202). For students whose storytelling began in the dramatizing mode, in which words do not carry the entire weight of responsibility for communicating the story, writing the story brings to the forefront the requirements of narrative structure and language. What may have been unconscious during the telling comes into awareness in the writing. In turn, what is fostered during writing brings clarity to the telling of subsequent stories. The teller learns to see how the imagined story fits into an overarching narrative frame. We will take a closer look at this process in the section on the graphic organizer in this chapter.

- *Impact of telling on the writer's ear:* 'You can edit your writing to make it *sound better* than your telling.'

  For these students, the sensory experience of telling the story to another person is a vital resource they take with them into the act of recording their stories. The story exists in the ear prior to writing – as it is told – and after writing – as it is retold. The structure, cadence, and intonation of the spoken words echo in auditory memory and support the writer as she 'replaces words with images of words' (Vygotsky 1934/1986, p.181). The sensory aspect of spoken story undergirds the writing.

## The prerequisite for freedom from anxiety

Writing happens when writers are not self-critical or tense, are free from fear.

> Learning that it was important to just get ideas out and not worry about waiting for the best idea helped get us started... Knowing not to worry about spelling or having the best vocabulary from the very beginning helped us get going... Knowing we can go back and bump up our writing, edit with each other and take out or improve our ideas helped us not get stuck... Basically, learning that all our ideas are important and it is okay to let them all fly out... It doesn't have to always be the best idea first.

I recall when I tried to golf for the first time. It was with colleagues, all avid golfers. Despite their understanding and patience, I felt myself becoming more and more inept. After a first good hit, it was a downward spiral – I, all powerless to help it. My anxiety, more than my inexperience, was the problem. Nine years old again and picked last for the baseball team. Krashen writes about this phenomenon when he describes how an 'affective filter' of anxiety can impede the process of learning a second language:

> If the acquirer is anxious...does not consider himself or herself to be a potential member of the group that speaks the language... he or she may understand the input but it will not reach the language acquisition device. The presence of the affective filter explains how two students can receive the same (comprehensible) input, yet one makes progress while the other does not. One student is open to the input while the other is not. (2003, p.6)

Like a gatekeeper, anxiety stands in the way of integrating new learning.

In reading the student comments, we can almost feel the collective sigh of relief breathed by writers who have walked into a wide-open space unhindered by debilitating anxiety regarding mistakes. The students in the end-of-year interview are reporting the gatekeeper to be off-duty. Self-criticism and fear of failure are replaced by serene trust in the sequence of the writing process ('it doesn't have to always be the best idea first'), the sense of support from the 'club' ('we can go back and edit with each other'), and self-confidence ('all our ideas are important').

## SCAFFOLDING SUPPORT FOR WRITERS

The pace of building/telling differs from that of recording. Completing the writing of a story can take many days. Students may return to a chosen story day after day, while continuing to build and tell about new and different worlds. The result is that the content of the writing does not always reflect the current tray, nor can it. Alternatively, students may continue to modify a particular world to effect the evolution of its story as they continue to process it in the sand and in the writing. In both cases, the recording of the chosen tale takes on a life of its own, reflecting the process of writing – draft, conference, revise, edit, and publish.

### Time frame of sandtray writers' workshop

A sandtray workshop that incorporates the writing component will require a time frame of approximately 90 minutes:

- *Greeting:* 5 minutes
- *Building:* 20–25 minutes
- *Partner sharing (storytelling and listening feedback):* 10–15 minutes
- *Gathering – mid-workshop mini-lesson and group sharing:* 10–15 minutes
- *Writing and peer conferencing:* 30 minutes
- *Cleanup and farewell:* 5–10 minutes

If your goal is to capitalize on the writing opportunity spawned from the activities of the first two segments, but a short workshop time precludes the possibility of a writing component, you can offer students the opportunity to record in a venue and time frame separate from building and oral storytelling. In that event, the techniques that function as links and memory prompts outlined in the subsequent sections become crucial.

## Linking building and telling to writing: Photograph, grid map, graphic organizer

Sandtray play has generated ideas; oral storytelling has put them into words. The student who is recording needs a way to recall, access, and organize what has already been produced and created. The photograph and the grid map serve as visual references to the sandworld and the story map as reminder and organizer of the story that has been told.

### *Photograph of sandworld*

Place a digital photograph of the completed sandworld on the student drive. When a student logs into his own drive, he can thereby access the visual record of the worlds he has made. The sand picture acts as a reminder of the told story and as a story prompt. These photographs can be placed online, opening up flexibility in access and response. For example, a world created in the withdrawal setting of the resource room can be accessed during a writers' workshop in the regular classroom.

### *Grid map*

Provide grid paper in order for students to map their worlds (Figure 6.1). Teach students to map shapes of the figures in the tray onto the grid in correspondence to their placement in the sandworld, and to incorporate symbols in connection with legends that define what they represent. This activity links with mapping skills taught in the social studies curriculum such as locating places on a grid, estimating distances using scale, understanding common map symbols, and creating map keys or legends.

The map acts as visual prompt and reminder for recording the story and develops visual-spatial sense. Because it employs a picture symbol system, the map might be considered an intermediate step to the alphabetic symbolization of letters and written words. It builds visual literacy (Figure 6.1).

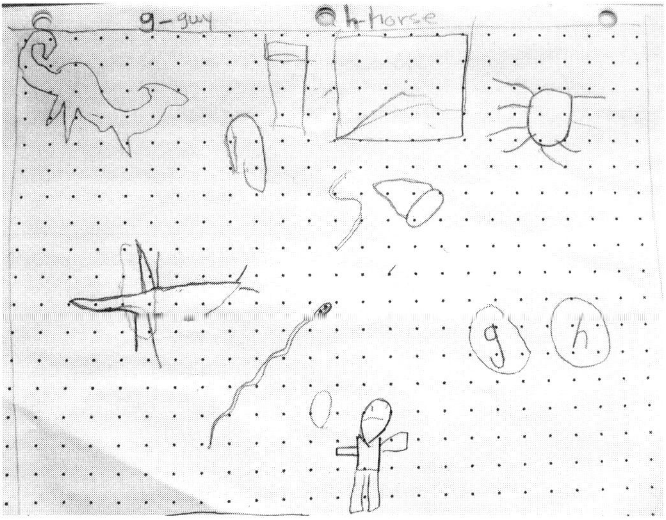


*Figure 6.1 Grid map, primary student*

## *Graphic organizer*

The graphic organizer (Figure 6.2) is a simple graphic that functions as both reminder and organizer for the sandtray storymaker. As a reminder, it cues students to the story they have told as they embark on writing it down. As an organizer, it builds familiarity with story components, orienting authors to the macrostructure of the narrative. Because it is a visual frame, it displays the relationship of narrative parts to the whole, arranging and categorizing them.

### Using the graphic organizer: 'But my story is like a jazz song'

A graphic organizer is a visual support that can be used at different junctures in the process of storymaking. When completed after building and preliminary to telling the story, the story map assists students in recollecting and ordering the ideas experienced through the hands-on play. It may be especially useful for students with short-term memory difficulties who struggle with accessing and ordering the story as they have envisioned it during the building of the world.

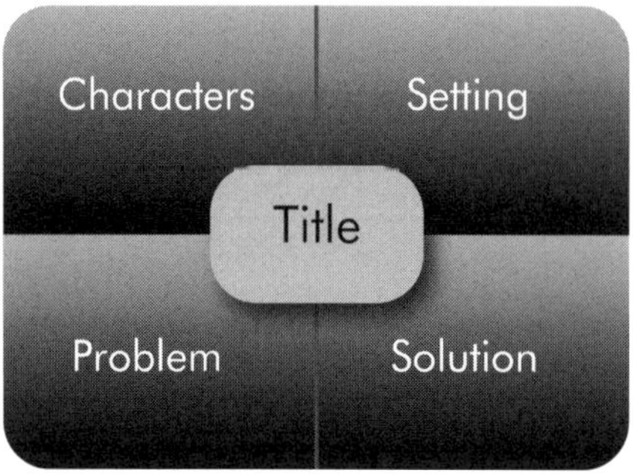


- Title is the central organizing principle
- Characters and Setting answer 'Who?' and 'Where?' 'When?'
- Problem or complicating action
- Solution answers 'How?'

*Figure 6.2 Simple graphic organizer*

But not all students find a benefit from mapping the story prior to telling it. One perceptive storyteller in Grade 6 (age 11) voiced his dissatisfaction with the technique when he said to Andrea Slocombe, 'But my story is like a jazz song. I don't know the plan until I have told it.' This student needs to explore where his story is going by speaking it out loud. Completing an organizer prior to the telling of the story would determine and delimit the story parameters before he could discover them.

Music making, as it turns out, may give us a very good image for understanding storymaking. *The Musical Brain*, a documentary video of Daniel Levitin's research, films Levitin using functional magnetic resonance imaging to reveal the brain activity of Sting as he composes an original melody (Pochmursky 2009). We see that while composing, the *corpus callosum* of the master musician is highly active, highly lit up. The *corpus callosum* is a bridge that links both sides of the brain, a neural highway that connects the right hemisphere, which is linked to emotion, with the left hemisphere, which is linked to cognition. Both sides, we see, are involved in music making. This can help us envision what happens in storymaking. The creative, emotional, inspired, inventive side informs the organizing, structuring side. And vice versa.

Both are necessary. The language of 'undirected thought' must relate to that of 'directed thought'. Students of story composition cannot ignore one aspect while focusing solely on the other.

Once he has discovered the story through the creative process of oral narration, the boy whose storytelling is 'like a jazz song' can slot the component parts of the story into the structure of the organizer. When he does sit down to categorize those elements in a visual display, he illuminates how all the parts of the story are connected, how they fit into the overall structure. At this juncture the story map does not determine or delimit the narrative, but helps the teller stand back from it and understand it, the better to write it down.

When completed after the telling, a graphic organizer arranges the narrative into an outline that will be referenced during recording. It functions as a tool that is in the service of the story, not as a straightjacket that shuts down the creative process. The story map is a guide to the teller-turned-author; its clarity advises the writing. The summary of problem and solution presents the direction of the plot; the listing of characters and setting display what the reader will need to know. In this way the organizer functions as compass and reference point for an author who is in the process of recording what she has already imagined and related.

### Introducing the graphic organizer

To familiarize students with the story map, deconstruct read-aloud stories with the group and summarize these stories in a visual art activity as follows:

- After the shared reading of a storybook, divide the class into four groups in order to map the story.
- Instruct each group to summarize one category (characters, setting, problem, or solution) through visual art such as cut and paste, paint, sketching, or drawing.
- Arrange the collection of the children's art in collages on the labeled quadrants of a large poster-sized sheet. Post on the workshop wall.

- The poster provides an organized visual retelling to which the students can refer when they are creating their own stories and story maps, and to which teachers can refer in mini-lessons about narrative structure.

When the students are making individual maps, instruct them first to title their story in the centre square and then to make quick sketches or outline in point form the characters, the setting, the problem, and solution, in the corresponding quadrants of the frame (Figure 6.3).

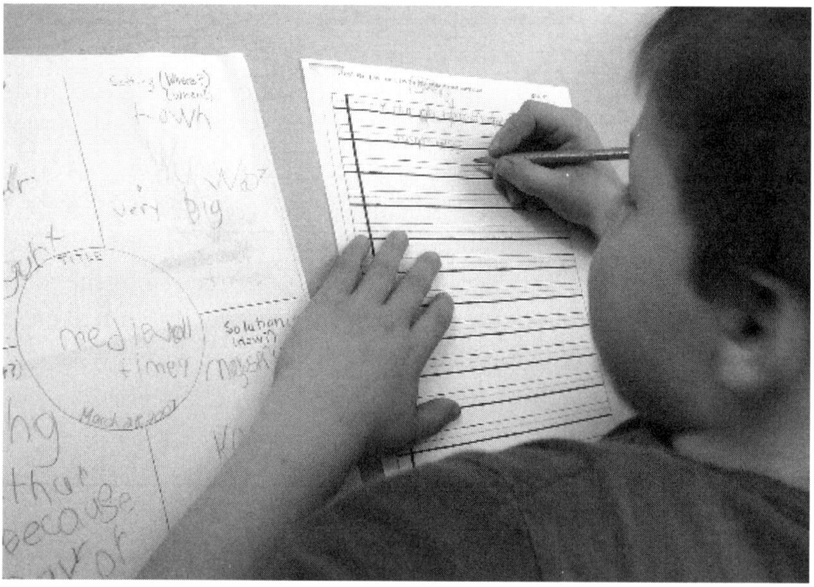

*Figure 6.3 Writing the story with story map support*

## Resources for lesson planning

Master teachers such as Lucy Calkins (2003) in her series *Units of Study for Primary Writing*, Nancie Atwell (2002) in *Lessons that Change Writers*, and Dorfman and Capelli (2007) in *Mentor Texts* are a few of the authors who have given us bodies of work that provide rich resources on lesson content, assessment, and evaluation for teachers of student writers across the years of elementary school. My intention in this section is not to reiterate what they have offered so inspiringly to teachers, but to refer you to their work. The pedagogy that they have developed is a seamless fit with the social and emotional goals of the sandtray narrative workshop. The 'author's celebration' is one example of this. Suggested by Calkins and Mermelstein (2003, p.115) as a way to showcase student writing by sharing published pieces on special days, the celebrations infuse the workshop with enthusiasm, add a further audience for the writing, and develop a sense of a community among the participants. In adapting the idea of the 'author celebration' to the resource room setting, I invited the wider classroom audience to hear the sandtray stories of the special education withdrawal group.

- On celebration days, which we called 'publishing parties', the visiting classroom population rotated in small groups to hear peers who had been withdrawn for sandtray play and storymaking read selected works that had undergone the cycle of draft, revision, and edit, and were now being presented in final 'published' version.
- The visiting classmates offered appreciations and questions. An adult who accompanied each group scribed the comments on cards, thus providing the authors with a written record of peer feedback. The cards were housed in envelopes for each author.
- Adapting Calkins and Mermelstein's suggestion, at the culmination of the celebration, the authors shared snacks and toasts with the classroom audience.
- The shared stories, along with the feedback cards, were showcased on a bulletin board in the hallway. Interested passers-by who stopped to read the stories were invited to add written comments and place them in the author's envelopes.
- The care with which the authors' work was stored, displayed, and celebrated conveyed to the students its importance.
- A further benefit was discovered. The writers invariably supplemented the reading of their stories by sharing with their classmates a description of the workshop activities. Their sharing produced an introduction and unveiling of sandtray play to classmates who had not participated. It demystified the

process and dissolved the sense of separateness that sometimes accompanies students in a withdrawal group. The description of the sandtray play was received with emotions akin to awe and envy – a gratifying response for participants in the resource group.

## VIOLENCE IN STORY CONTENT

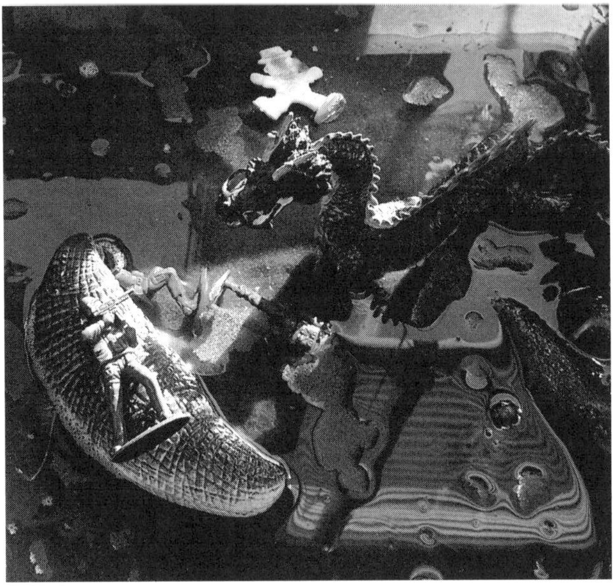

*Figure 6.4 Dragon slayer*

As they do in the building of their worlds, sandplayers often express aggression, hostility, ferocity, bloodshed, and struggle in their storywriting. It is not our task to try to prevent violence or fearful situations from showing up in student stories; instead, our task is to teach our storymakers to situate these within a frame of meaning. The fact is, violence by itself is not sufficient. Gratuitous violence belongs to the video game; it does not make a satisfying story. An author needs to show how conflict makes a character feel, how conflict makes a character change and grow.

Classic stories, including fairy tales and myths such as the tale of St. George and the Dragon reinvented by the maker of the world of Figure 6.4, are stories about threshold barriers.[1] In these stories, the path the character takes leads him into struggle and often into bloodshed. The hero encounters a barrier; faces it; and, by facing it, grows. Not by evading the battle, but by defying the enemy, is the character changed. Only by confrontation of the obstacle, often with necessary violence and requisite aggression, does he overcome.

Meaningful and necessary conflict in service of the story is what we want to challenge our students to describe. Enlist the classic tales. Demonstrate how conflict is connected to character development by choosing shared reading stories of threshold barriers. These stories provide an alternative to the one-dimensional video game model of violence that often informs the sensibility of our students. Bettelheim writes that children need to hear real fairy tales even though such stories can be frightening or gruesome, and he warns against giving them to children in 'prettified and simplified versions which subdue their meaning and rob them of all deeper significance' (1977, p.24). Read aloud to students unabridged fairy tales and stories that contain fearful situations such as *Sylvester and the Magic Pebble* (Steig 1969), literature such as *The Hobbit* (Tolkien 1986), the ancient story of *Gilgamesh* (Zeman 1995), and myths such as St. George and the Dragon. These texts contain violence and fearful situations that are in the service of the story and the character's development, and resonate as meaningful to the hearer.

## EXAMPLES OF STORY SERIES

It is difficult to imagine the story series included in this section ever arising out of a sentence starter or teacher-assigned topic writing. Students who have done symbol play in the sand typically write stories that wrestle with struggles near to their hearts. Writing that arises from sandtray play is often similar to the writing that is engendered

---

1 My thanks to Vicky Mathies for insights gained in our conversations about threshold barriers and the role of the shared reading of classic literature in demonstrating to students how to integrate violence in their writing.

by guided imagery exercises, described by Allan and Bertoia in *Written Paths to Healing* as holding 'images that reflect wounding, healing or core psychological struggles' (1992, p.191). They note that writing helps children who have experienced trauma 'think through and reflect on experience, which can result in a new understanding and a feeling of control which at times leads to a sense of empowerment' (p.124).

Sometimes the story discloses innovative possibilities for solving real-life dilemmas. The playful work in the tray, and the storymaking that derives from it, can open up new approaches to intractable problems. The story functions as an intermediate space in which the maker can try and discard – or keep and develop – possible treatments of the plots that engross him. The imagination, Harold Clarke Goddard proffers in his commentary on William Blake, can 'uncreate evil' (1956, p.35).

In each of the following four examples we see a child addressing important themes over a series of consecutive stories. The four series demonstrate that, given the right conditions, a child will externalize and work out inner confusions that insistently demand a voice. In the arc of these sandworld narratives we can see that children work with the same questions, day after day, either until they have exhausted their resources in dealing with the issue, or until they find a resolution to their perplexity and are satisfied. The questions pondered in the following series are, respectively: How does reconciliation occur? What is a family? Who will be in charge? How do I belong?

## 1. The conflict series (*How does reconciliation occur?*)

In the following example, the stories are a series of riffs on a single plot line, a single problem. The early primary-age student is reiterating over and over again in a variety of settings and circumstances the situation in which characters impulsively lose control, fight or hurt one another, and apologize. The writer does not introduce any strategy or tool for dealing with the aftermath of conflict beyond that which is introduced in the initial story: 'Say sorry'. Perhaps in this series the child is saying that she has found conflict to be inevitable, but is reassuring herself that conflict is not the end of the world; the relationship disrupted by her impulsivity can be healed with an apology.

- (December 8): First thare wus a land. Then a rinoe had a flag. He put it in the grownd. Then a snake came. He wanted it too. They where mad. They where fiteing. So bad... Oh No! The rinoe wus hurt. Then the snake said sorry to the rineoe. The end.
- (December 10): Frst there wus a bear. It's name wus King Z. He had sum kusin's. Then they had to fite. Oh no... The Bear wus MAD. He did not wont to fite. But he had to. Then he got mad. Problum... He got SO mad that he nockt them out. He whus sorey. He sed sory a kupl times. Then he ment it. The end.
- (December 14): First ther whus a wulf and a polr ber. He wus mad! HE PUNCHT THE WULF. OH NO...THE WULF WUS HRT. I AM SORY. I AM SORY.
- (December 15): First there wus sum anamuls. They where happy. Oh Lookit. There is that new anamull. He wus happy too. Then the dinosaur sed helloe! They did a meen thing. They did not sae aneething. Then he sed nothing bak. Instead...He...wopt them over! I am sory I am sory. Wud you wont to have a party.
- (January 8): *The Queen.* The Queen is mad. She wons to have a husbind. Then she made a fite. Yes! Said a man. Yes! Yes! Yes! Said a nethr man. Whel see! said the Queen. It is a Oh No! I am sorry! I am sorry!
- (January 14): *The Animals.* There are sum sea creechers. They live in the ocean. It is fun. Oh no! One of the sea creachers was hurt biy a nothr creacher. 'Oh no! I am sorry! I ment to hit the shark!'
- (February 5): *The Day.* One day a king and a queen they love to play together. Then one day they hade a fite. They puncht and kickd. It was not fun. Then they said sorry to echuther.

## 2. The castle series (*How do the king and queen relate?*)

In the following series, written over a time frame of approximately two months, the child is working out the story of the relationship between the king and the queen. The writing helps the child reflect upon the forces that the king and queen symbolize. Whether these are players in the child's psyche or symbolic representations of the child's actual father and mother we do not know. Nor do we need to know. The child is working out his own question in sand and in storymaking. The link between the first six stories is emphasized by the author's designation of them as chapters. The series ends finally with a resolution, reminiscent of a fairy tale ending with the drawing of a castle evenly balanced by turrets and flags and with the words, 'Then they lived together and were happy' (Figure 6.5).

---

- *Chapter 1:* Once upon a time there was a King and a Queen. It was fun. They went to a shop. They bot sum stuff. They whr rich. They eevin had a limo. They eevin had a tiger. He was the guard tiger. He was fun too. He wuod growl at the intruders. The King and the Queen whr talking bout the tiger. Then the tigert hrd sumthing about him. He only heard them saying bad things even though they were saying good things too. Then the tiger ran away. The King and Queen lukd and lukt. But...they did not see him. Then they got in the limo and then they lukt and lukt. But...then they saw him. With the binokulars. They whr happy. And the tiger was happy too.
- *Chapter 2:* Then all of the tigers and the cheetahs ran away. They wher happy. When the Queen and the King saw that the anamals wher gon... 'OH NO.' They wher sad, Where are they? Then they came home. The End
- *Chapter 3: The King's Problum.* First there wus a King and a Queen. They whr happy. They wher having fun to. Then they whent home. 'OH NO!' The house is a mes. Ye thot? Then they cleend up. The End
- *Chapter 4: A King and a Queen.* First ther wus a King and a Queen. It wus fun. They went to the beach. They went

around town. They stopped at stores and they bought stuff. But…they had to go home. But they did not wont to go home. But they went home.

- *Chapter 5: A King and a Queen.* First the King wus out and he wus not doing wut he wus suposet do. And the Queen. and she wus at home cleening up. It was rilly boring. Then she fond the King. You need to cum home. *The End of the ho in tire book.*
- *Chapter 6: The Queen and The King.* The Queen was happy. Then something hapind. Her castle was falling down. 'Oh NO!' she said. Then the King fixed the castle. The Queen and the King. The End
- *The King and the Queen.* Ther where a King and a Queen and there son named Z and a noos reporter. First there was a King and a queen and the son. The lived in a casul. It was fun. Then the noos ruportr came biy. He mist our casl! Then she saw our casl. Thank you noos ruportr! The End
- *King and Queen.* The King loved kids! And the queen loved kids too! And of course they Love each other. The King had a limo. The queen had a limo too. They even had dirt bikes. 'Hi,' said the King to the boy. 'Hi,' said the queen to the girl. 'I love kids,' said the King and the Queen! They live in a castle. 'I love our castle,' said the King. 'I Love the castle too!' said the Queen. The King and the Queen wanted a bigger castle. They need a bigger castle, too. 'I wish we had a bigger castle!' Then the King and the queen bilt a big castle. And they loved kids even more. And they loved each other even more too. They had cool things too.
- *The Fite.* First there was a queen. She had a friend. Then she wantid the king's people. He wantid her frends to. Then they lived together. And they whr happy. The End. (see Figure 6.5)

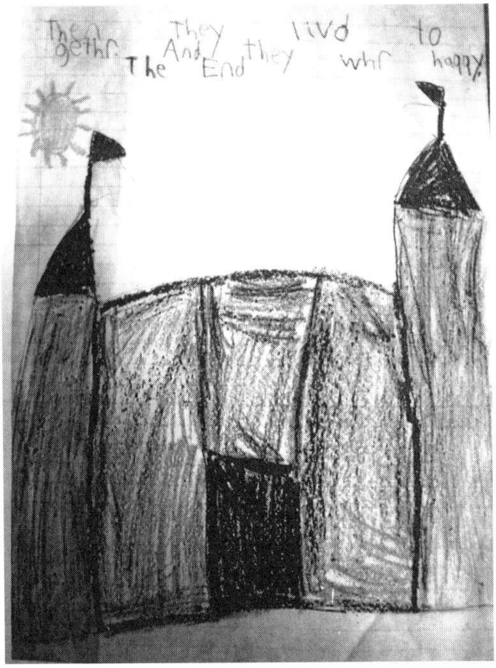


*Figure 6.5 'Then they livd together. And they whr happy. The End.'*

## 3. The authority series (*Who will be in charge?*)

In the following series, written in the two-week interval between May 28 and June 12, the student repeats the scenario of the death of a king and his replacement ('The king is dead, long live the king'). Is he trying to reflect on the vagaries of the schoolyard politics, the jockeying for positions of dominance? Are the stories an expression of the warring elements in his psyche? Is he trying to figure out who is the authority in his life? Is he puzzling about the permanence of death? We do not know. What does seem clear is that he is working out, day after day, one question that rests in the forefront of his mind.

- *The King Tiger* (May 28) Once upon a time a Tiger was a King! He ate the King! So the tiger ate the King of pepelle, so what! He was hungry and the King was the only person around. But it was fun. The End

- *The King Egell* (May 29) Once upon a time...a egell ate the king. It was not alawd. But...the egell did eat the King. It was sad and they had a funerl for the King. But...now the egell was in charge. And the egell did whut he wanted. Now the egell was happy to be the King. the End
- *The King Bare* (May 30) Once upon a time a bare was in the wuds and his bruthr egell was there too! They did not like each uthr. They hated each uthr. The bare started a fiyt. 'Bring it on!' said the bare. 'No' said the egell. 'Yes' said the Bare. 'OK' said the egell. Then they had a fite. Then the egell was ded. The End
- *The King Egell* (May 31) OK you now know the story of the King Bare, rite? OK, well I'll let you in on a little seakret. The King egell is *not* ded. The King Bare made him alive, ok! The egell is alive and he is the King agen! 'Wow' said the vilig. And...th King egell ate the King Bare.
- *King Gren* (June 1) Once upon a time King Gren is now ded because he was in a fite. It was sad. They had a funrl for King Gren. Then King Gren went to the hospitl. They cant do anything ther. Then they put him in his chambr. Then he was alive agen.
- *The King Bird* (June 5) We will get another king tomorrow. But we have King...Bird! He is famous, yah. King Bird was sik, 'Oh no can you help him?' 'Mabee but we don't know for shur!' 'No we can not!' 'But let him on his own, okay.' 'Okay' Then one morning... 'He is alive!' 'Yes I told you!' *It is good to be the King!* The End
- *The King Frog* (June 6) The King Frog is ded because the TReks kild him! 'Put him in his chambr.' 'Yes Sir!' That night...POW. The King is alive agen, '*Yes!*'
- *The Prince Snake* (June 7) Once upon a time there was a celebration and the peepll that where invited did not...cum. 'Oh NO how can we get thare!' BRrring BRrring BRrring BRrring 'Hello!' 'Hello!' We filmed the celebration!' 'Yes!' 'Cen you send it' 'Yes we cen. But...it will take...hmmm... let me see the calindr... It will take a week? 'OK.' THE END

## 4. The friendship series (*How do I belong?*)

The author of the following three stories below was a sensitive introverted child whose stated intention was to be a writer. She began the year with an aversion to the hurly-burly of the classroom. A specially trained worker had gradually acclimatized her to longer and longer days at school. Her stories, even at age seven, had the sophistication of the avid reader and dreamer. In her work in the sandtray and storymaking, begun part way through the school year, she reflected upon her situation from the safe vantage point of the imagination. The initial three stories of her sandtray workshop experience are reproduced here. They are, I think, asking the question 'How do I belong?' It is clear that in this short window of time she moved from confusion to clarity and, in the last story, reached a possible resolution.

---

- *Story 1: The Magic Kingdom:* There wonets was a magic kingdom and everything was going a little too crazy. There was a cat named Frizly and he pownst on a magic snake and then he fell asleep. And the queen of all sea cretures ws taking over the kingdom. Some guys are hunting down a dinesore. ROOOR saud the dinesore and the sea food guys where in a car and hunting a clam crab to eat for his sea food.

- *Story 2: Sosen is Lost:* There was a little girl named Sosen and she was all alone in the jungle, lost and scared. There was a snake slithering along and he said to Sosen, 'What's the matter?' 'I'm lost, I'm cold, I'm scared. I can't take it,' cried Sosen as she sat by her tent. 'SISSSSSSSSISSSS' said the snake. So Sosen walked in the forest farther and suddenly RRRRORRRR. What can it be? It is a lion. AAAA said Sosen as she ran behind a big tree.

  'Its ok, little girl,' said the lion. 'What is the matter?'
  'I'm lost, I'm cold, I'm scared,' said Sosen.
  'It's okay,' said the lion.
  'You are not that scary,' said Sosen.
  'Why did you think I was?' said the lion.

- *Story 3: A Girl in Need;* Once upon a time there were lots of trees and animals. There was a girl named Kayla and she was not an ordinary girl she was so nice. But she wanted to help people. So she saw Nony and she was sitting on a rock so she went to talk to her and she said, 'Can I help you?'

  'No,' said Nony.

  'OK,' said Kayla and then she saw Ron sitting down. 'Can I help you?'

  'No,' said Ron.

  'Okay,' said Kayla.

  Then she saw Moose. 'Hello Moose,' she said. 'Can I help you?'

  'NO,' said Moose.

  'All I want is to help. Why can't anyone understand me?'

  'We do but we're bizey.'

  Do you want to play now? Said Kayla.

  Yes said the animals. Let's play. Yay said Kayla and they played and played and played and played all day long.

  And that's the end.

## Chapter 7

# STORIES FROM SANDWORLD CLASSROOMS

*'My brain is always ready in here.'*

– Jeremy, Grade 5 (age 10) sandtray narrative workshop student

*'Where we got to go had treasure.'*

– Michael, Grade 6 (age 12)

Word of mouth in a collegial school spreads quickly. A positive contagion. The experiment that began with the small group of Grade 2 (age seven) students was replicated as we discovered that the simple procedure of finding ideas through the sandplay and expressing them in the words of story was a portable one, adaptable to different contexts, a moveable feast. Teachers in the school experimented with their own adaptations in small-group and whole-class settings. Frequency and duration varied – daily, weekly, bi-weekly, in eight-week blocks, or for the entire school year, with entire classes or with withdrawal groups. Some situations offered the hands-on and storytelling components, while others extended to storywriting. This chapter will tell some stories of these classrooms: stories from my resource room as well as from the classrooms of Jane Keevil, Christopher Kemp, Cheryl Schmid, and Andrea Slocombe.

## SOCIAL SKILLS GROUPS

Empathy training, anger management, and impulse control are the common business of social skills groups – small groups intensively focused on the social-emotional curriculum. Members of these groups are predominantly students who need modeling and rehearsal of replacement behaviours for aggression and bullying, training in emotional awareness, and an immersion in respectful listening (Cefai and Cooper 2009). The school introduced sandtray play to these groups both as an undirected activity, in which sand and miniatures were provided and the children were left to determine what they would build next (examples 1 and 2), and in a directed activity, in which the teacher assigned a specific scenario to the students to build in the sand (examples 3 and 4).

## 1. Grade 6 (age 11) boys group

Grade 6 (age 11) is a year of transition; adolescence is just around the corner. For boys facing challenges such as attention deficit disorder, a learning disability, an intellectual delay, or Asperger's, or who are recovering from a trauma, this year can be crucial. Six boys who were coping with some of these challenges formed a weekly 45-minute sandtray play narrative group.

- In the sharing that followed the individual greeting and building, the entire group rotated to hear the story of each tray. The boys themselves drove this decision, stating that they wanted the cohesion that group sharing fostered. The additional benefit was that teacher prompting and modeling of listening responses could take place with the whole group.
- Each week the boys mapped their worlds onto graph paper, the placement and details of characters and setting recorded by means of grids and the legends they devised. These maps went with them back to class.
- During the workshop, photographs were taken of their sandworlds, which the boys accessed on the school's computer system in their individual student drives. Because both map and photographs were available in their classroom, the boys were able to follow up with recording in the context of the writing block within the regular programming. Together, the map and photographic record created a planner for narrative writing.

- The photographic record of the worlds meant that at the end of the term, the boys were able to create movies of their stories.

### *What worked*

The opportunity for creative play and hands-on activity in their late childhood sparked the enthusiasm of each of the participants. A number of the boys told me that this 45-minute period was the highlight of their week. Confronting a wide variety of challenging life situations, the boys gave time and space to issues that were close to their hearts, coming back week after week to the same themes. Every one of the group members grew in their storytelling and listening capabilities.

Although the group varied widely in individual strengths and needs, there were no social divisions observable during the workshop. The demand to offer thoughtful feedback created an immersion in the practice of kindness. The boys were highly enthusiastic about each others' worlds, their questioning and feedback evidence of their interest in each others' stories. They adopted an attitude of supportiveness to one another. The group fostered friendships that carried over into classroom and playground.

## 2. Recess clubs and before-school clubs

Recess clubs and before-school clubs provided an alternative recess setting for students who were having severe social difficulties on the playground. This play took place within the resource room with the special education resource teacher.

- Students built a world, told the story, and gave feedback to one another.
- Within the small group, the teacher modeled and coached skills in listening and giving appropriate feedback.

### *What worked*

As one component of a menu of activities, sandtray play provided an opportunity for students in the recess clubs to build skills needed for reintegration on the playground. Within their enthusiasm for the play, students experienced the opportunity to decompress, develop facility with narrative structure, give and receive positive feedback, and build friendships.

The before-school clubs were a calming introduction to the school day for students who arrived off the school bus in the morning in an agitated state. Salvaging what formerly had been a dead space in the day before the bell rang, the clubs facilitated transition to the classroom. Sandplay in a quiet space was a centring activity. The play itself allowed expression of issues and emotions that clamoured for a voice.

## 3. Debriefing from behaviour incident

In this use of sandplay, children deconstructed and reconstructed in the tray an incident after an altercation or misbehaviour. Sandplay was used here in a directed way. The sandtray was used as a tool to help the student step back from the incident in order to take the measure of justified responsibility for it and to determine how to handle a similar situation in future. The exercise also opened the way for a discussion about making amends. The student was instructed to build two sandtray scenes in order to elicit a two-part reflection:

- *The first tray:* What actually happened? In building the first tray, the student showed what happened and articulated the narrative of the incident. The tray was dismantled and the student asked to build a second tray.
- *The second tray:* What will I do next time? The building of a second tray gave the child a way to make a new storyline. The narrative developed in the second tray was then written down in the form of a plan. It was the child's stated intention for coping with a similar situation in the future and was signed by the child.

### *What worked*

The activity of reproducing in the sand of the first tray the incident as it had transpired was a grounding work. The tray functioned as a non-threatening locale in which the scenario could be replayed and seen again from a safe distance. Because it gave the child space to express and externalize the feelings elicited by the incident, it helped her return to an emotional equilibrium. Dismantling the first tray was a way of removing the incident into the past.

The second tray made use of hands-on imagination as the child envisioned and built a new world in which she determined an alternate way of responding to a similar situation in future. She did this not out of lip service to expected norms, but out of the freedom of individual creativity. The child was no longer in defensive mode, the teacher no longer in lecturing mode.

Sandplay gave children a way of seeing the event from the perspectives of the different players. It did this literally, as they placed the figures in the tray. Because of this, it became a springboard for discussion about student commitments to make amends to anyone who had been affected by the incident. The world in the tray informed the subsequent discussion.

Finally, with the writing (or, in the case of very young children, the scribing) and signing of a behaviour plan arising out of the building of a second world, a real accountability was invoked. With a record made of his intentions, the child was answerable.

This use of sandtray play in a directed way opened the way for the teacher to engage in an invitational manner with the process of discipline described by Colorosa as 'Show children what they have done wrong; give them ownership of the problem; help them find ways of solving the problem; leave their dignity intact' (2002, p.79).

## 4. Mixed-age (kindergarten to Grade 5 (age ten)) social skills group

Five students, ranging in age from kindergarten to Grade 5 (age 10), met together in a group twice weekly for 25 minutes in an adaptation of sandtray play targeting their aggression and social difficulties.

- The teacher asked the group members to build a world that 'showed kids being friends'. Students were instructed about the theme of their worlds and the discussion. The discussion of the worlds was framed by questions that provided opportunity for social skills coaching:
    - What do you think they did in the world that went wrong?
    - Show me what the character could have done.
    - What could the character say to the one he is fighting?
    - What might he do?
- The students elicited problem scenarios in individual sandtray play.
- They shared their worlds and the group came up with comments on how the problem in the worlds might be solved, providing suggestions to the teller for alternate endings that would solve the problems of the situation. The story became the basis for discussion about friendship skills.

### *What worked*

The physical playing-out of story scenarios gave the children a venue within which to rehearse and master difficult social situations. The peers themselves evaluated the scenarios and made suggestions. This kind of peer input was called by one teacher the 'power of the circle' to listen and give feedback. It was the mentorship of peers, a lived experience of social support, and a rehearsal of an alternative way of reacting that combined to make this a useful program.

There was definite measurable change in the behaviour of each of the group members as the year progressed, with significant gains in self-control, self-regulation, and anger management on the schoolyard. The end of the school year saw allotment for educational assistant support for two of the students reduced by 75 per cent.

## SANDTRAY PLAY AND STORYMAKING WITHIN THE MAINSTREAM CLASSROOM

A number of teachers found sandtray narrative play to be a viable program outside its niche as a 'special education activity'. Offered within the context of the regular classroom, it provides the benefit of imaginative, hands-on, play-based activity to mainstream students, demonstrating the validity of the catch phrase 'necessary for some, good for all'. Sandtray play can be incorporated in a variety of ways within the curriculum, at a variety of grade levels, as we see in the following examples.

### Storymaking stations: Junior and senior kindergarten

As seen in Chapter 4, developing the ability to frame and sequence narrative is a tool for the development of oral language in young children and may be characterized as a stepping stone to literacy. In Jane Keevil's junior/senior kindergarten class, a program that she called 'Storytelling Booths' delivered an opportunity for the development of oral storytelling for her kindergarteners. The storymaking activities fostered listening and responding, free exploration, independent application of their knowledge of story structure, and generalization of prior knowledge to make connections in a new situation.

- *Frequency and duration:* One hour daily for two-week blocks; the first block was offered during the fourth month, the second during the ninth month of the school year.
- Children rotated daily through stations: sandtrays, puppet theatre, felt boards, barn, castle, garage, police station, and logs.
- At their station of the day, children:
    - co-created a story in the play by making the scene
    - told the story together to a listening adult
    - made a drawing of the scene.

- *First rotation:* The initial storymaking rotation during the fourth month of school focused on the characters and setting. The children were instructed as follows:
    - build a world
    - tell the story of your world to the adult when she comes to your booth
    - draw the people in your world (characters) and where it happens (setting).
- *Preparation for second rotation:* Between the first rotation in the fourth month and the second in the ninth month, the children were introduced to the frame of 'Somebody... Wanted... But... So...' (Beers 2003, p.144). Jane discussed this in the context of many shared reading texts in order to familiarize the children with it.
- *Second rotation:* When the storymaking stations activity was repeated in the ninth month of school, Jane expanded the focus to include a plot line. The instructions to the children were:
    - build a world
    - tell your story to the adult using the starter words: *Somebody... Wanted... But... So...*
    - draw the most exciting part of the action.

### *What worked*

One morning as a guest in the kindergarten during the 'storytelling booths', I saw pairings of children dotted over the room, bent intently over their play/work. At one sandtray station I watched two students in their imaginative play:

> 'There is a fire at Santa's house. I have to rescue all the reindeers.' (*Raoul moved the deer.*) 'Then I have to take all the buildings away so they are safe.' (*He moved the entire setting to the other end of the tray.*)

> 'Now we are making a new world for the reindeer.' (*He began to create a new world at the opposite side.*)

Raoul's partner was completely absorbed in his story. As he continued to expand the plot, she went over to her paper and markers and began to draw the pictures of the reindeer. The two continued, deeply engrossed and oblivious to a succession of witnesses, including the school principal. Raoul, a student who had been receiving intensive intervention because of a language delay, was the creative director. Engaged in a play situation with a partner whose reading and writing skills were above average, he was nonetheless the leader, providing initiative with the storyline. His partner assigned for herself the role of recorder. This scenario was repeated again all over the kindergarten class. Children in mixed-ability pairings were absorbed in the exhilarating activity of imaginative play as their individual strengths were engaged and language skills in story sequencing and organization developed.

## Sandtray play in social studies

In Ontario, students in Grade 3 (age eight) and 4 (age nine) learn about some of the special features of the adaptations of plants and animals within their own habitats. Cheryl Schmid presented this content with a group of students using the medium of sandtray play and letter writing:

- Cheryl presented an overview of many habitats to her students and invited each to choose one habitat about which they wanted to become an expert.
- With materials specific to each habitat that Cheryl had provided for them, they replicated the habitat they had researched in the sandtray.
- They told the story of their tray to a partner.
- The partner listened and responded with two appreciations and a question.
- This routine of researching, building, and sharing orally was entrenched over the span of a few weeks.

- Inspired by the shared reading of *Meerkat Mail* (Gravett 2007), the students made an imaginative leap, taking on the identity of one creature within their own habitats.
- The students themselves sparked the evolution of the next development in the learning process. They decided that they were curious about the habitats of their peers and wanted to 'travel' to them. Letter writing began – letters to the inhabitants of different worlds with questions about that world. Scorpion decided to visit Horse, for example. An exchange of letters ensued. The writer asked questions about the recipient's world; the reply offered suggestions on what was needed to adapt to the unfamiliar habitat if they were to visit. Cheryl wrote to the students as well, modeling the questions and letter-writing format.

### *What worked*

Humour. The students entered a long-term role play in which imagination and lightness lent a playful synergy to the learning, effecting outcomes of increased knowledge and skills and improved attitudes. Building, oral sharing, letter writing, and communication among all the members of the group defined a project that evolved over many weeks. The layer of imaginative life established a whimsical connection between classroom members. Students were enthusiastic. Previously reluctant writers were engaged because the writing was in service to the interactions within the class and to the desire to share. Writing output and quality of writing increased.

## Whole-class use of sandtray play in the primary division

In some mainstream classes, sandtray play and storymaking was offered as a literacy station, open to small groups of students on a rotating basis. In other classrooms, it was offered as a whole class activity engaging all students simultaneously.

### Small-group literacy stations

During 40 minutes of the literacy block in which some students were engaged in guided reading groups, and the rest of the class at literacy stations, a storymaking station was offered as a choice for students in various primary classrooms. Four sandtrays and four bags of miniatures were made available. Over the week everyone in the class would rotate through the sandtray station. Students built a world and recorded the story on frames of setting, characters, problem, solution. They were given the opportunity to share their stories orally to the whole class at the culminating whole-group sharing time that concluded the literacy block. Evaluation was based on engagement, focus, accountability, and completed story frames. Use of on-task behaviours was tracked.

### What worked

The teachers who offered this station discovered that the students using it were focused and engaged. Students worked independently because of the inherently captivating nature of the sandtray play. Students keenly looked forward to their turn at the sandtray storymaking station. One teacher remarked that an intuitive next step would be to incorporate into the literacy block a storywriting station to follow the sandtray activity.

### Whole class

A level of organization and classroom management are required to run an effective sandtray narrative workshop with an entire class at one time. Christopher Kemp maintains that the key to success in doing this is careful preparation of the students and rehearsal of specific workshop behaviours.

- In order to train an entire class to approach the individual workspaces as places of solitude, Christopher set up two weeks at the outset of the school year in which every aspect of the workshop – building, telling, listening, recording, and cleanup – was modeled and explicitly taught. The class developed success criteria for each component of the workshop, created rubrics, and practised each skill separately.

- Christopher familiarized his students with the visual cue of 'QUIET' and a 'noise barometer' scaled for volume recognition. The result was that he could cue the students simply by pointing silently to either the 'QUIET' sign or the noise level on the barometer.
- It was important to establish a predictable routine for beginning the workshop. Upon entering the classroom, each student retrieved his own labeled sandtray and picked up a bag of miniatures at random. No sharing or trading of miniatures was allowed. The purpose of this was to seal the enclosure of quiet around the building time.

### *As calming activity*

Whole-class sandtray play and storytelling was used as a de-escalating strategy. Appropriating Ashton-Warner's phrase, as discussed in Chapter 1, Christopher referred to this activity as the 'breathing out' time for his students because it functioned as a centring and calming time at midday, after the children returned from their noon recess. The students built worlds individually and shared their stories in dyads. There was ongoing modeling of listening and responding to stories on alternate Fridays when the whole class met together for group sharing and responding to stories. This afforded ongoing opportunities for teacher-directed modeling of telling, questioning, and appreciating.

### *What worked*

The practice contributed to the sense of the class as a safe and welcoming place. For students who struggled emotionally, socially, or academically, it provided a needed play interlude in the school day, and resulted in a reduction in the number of outside interventions for behaviour needs.

### *As catalyst to narrative writing*

At specified times during the school year, when the class was focusing on narrative writing, Christopher incorporated a three-week sandtray play and storywriting component into the literacy block. Because the Grade 1 (age six) and 2 (age seven) students were unable to remember their sandtray stories over the two-day weekend break, Christopher incorporated a Monday-to-Friday pattern approximately as follows:

- *Monday:* The storyworlds were built in the sand. At the end of the session, the worlds were left intact. In succeeding days, the intact worlds were returned to student workspaces and used as a cue to trigger students' memories of the fullness of the stories they had imagined. Day by day, students were free to adjust the tray and develop the written story, changing details as the story evolved.
- *Tuesday:* Partner sharing and response to told stories of the sandworlds.
- *Wednesday:* Students made an outline of their stories on a 'Characters, setting, problem, solution' story organizer.
- *Thursday:* Students wrote the narrative using the planner they had completed on Wednesday.
- *Friday:* Whole-class sharing and celebration of stories.

### *What worked*

The storytelling fostered oral language development, both speaking and listening. When using the sandtray play as a catalyst for narrative writing, Christopher saw the play both as creating enthusiasm for storywriting as well as the mechanism by which his students generated ideas and organized them. The success of the sandtray program was evidenced by the fact that Christopher offered it for the three consecutive years that he taught early primary students.

## SPECIAL EDUCATION WITHDRAWAL GROUP: JUNIOR BOYS LITERACY

If you were to walk into Andrea Slocombe's resource room any time between 8.45 and 10.25 a.m. on any day of the week during the years of the experiment described in this section, you would have seen a group of eight boys from ages nine to thirteen engaged in the creation of story. A quick look around the interior of the classroom would have shown you there were eight designated areas outfitted with a sandtray and a bag of miniatures, a computer for each student, a gathering area with couch and chairs, and an interactive whiteboard that projected sandtray pictures and stories for group work. A variety of posters displayed key learning and student work, such as the one on telling the story:

Storytelling

- Ideas (get through sandplay)
- 'Wow' words
- Speak clearly
- Get to the point
- Grab people's attention
- Organize.

A whiteboard with 'Today's goals' had each boy's name and his stated goal. Among the list you might have seen one day were the individual goals: *I don't want my story to go on and on and I want to pause less... I want to speak louder and clearer... I want to explain more details in my characters... I want to add more details when describing the setting.*

Depending on the week's focus, you would have found at each student's office a self- or peer-evaluation sheet such as the one shown in Figure 7.1.

## Set-up

- The workshop followed the pattern of individual entry, build, tell, gather, and record.
- New learning was supported with a mid-workshop gathering for Brain Gym® (see Chapter 2) and a mini-lesson on aspects of storytelling, listening, and writing.

- The boys received direct instruction in effective use of technology with the intent that they would become independent writers, growing beyond the need for dictating their thoughts to a scribe, their writing becoming a full and satisfying expression of their thinking. They became conversant in various Ministry of Education owned programs and assistive technology. They accessed various websites that gave the students opportunity to illustrate and animate their writing.

Oral language peer assessment…just the beginning!

Name ____________ Partner's name ____________

| My partner… | ☑☑ | ☑ | Not yet! |
|---|---|---|---|
| Introduced the characters at the beginning of the story | | | |
| Had a beginning that describes the setting | | | |
| Told the beginning so that it created a picture in my mind | | | |
| Used words to describe the action of the story | | | |
| Spoke with good volume | | | |

*Figure 7.1 Peer evaluation sheet: Telling*

## Evaluation

The students' Ontario Writing Assessment scores and reading scores were tracked. Portfolios of student work were maintained. The students completed attitude and interest surveys and self-reflections at the outset and the conclusion of each term, filling in a rating scale that dealt with issues such as engagement in literacy, attentiveness, effort, behaviour, and competence connected with literacy tasks, attitude, and enjoyment of school.

## Outcome

A look at the before- and after-workshop data collection is eloquent affirmation of the usefulness of the program. Samples of the participants' writing skills were taken at the beginning of the program and at intervals throughout the program. Students whose writing scores in formal assessment had been at least two grades behind those of their peers demonstrated accelerated growth within four months. Province-wide testing for reading and writing was administered at the outset of the program and at end-of-year. At end-of-year, each boy completed the testing with total independence. No more scribing for these students: they used their word processors. Students who had been demonstrating behaviour difficulties and poor social skills and who had been struggling to generate ideas in the classroom showed significant improvements in all areas. Repeatedly, teacher and student scales rating skills and attitudes showed growth to 8 or 9 from an initial score of 0 to 2.

### *What worked*

Just four months into the project, the students' self-reports bore witness to a profound shift in the way they were approaching school. Comments from September such as 'I hate writing' were replaced with the comments that follow. Taking a closer look at what the students said, we can learn what worked for them and why:

1. Skills gained in the intensive setting generalized to classroom: *Now I don't have to sit in class trying to do something I can't do. I can*

*write or talk about my idea... I like what I am doing in literacy now. I don't get bored...*

2. Writing competency was fast-tracked: *I have really advanced in my writing. In September I could write one line in an hour and now* [four months later] *I can write four paragraphs maybe more...*

3. Frustration with writing tasks and the behaviours stemming from frustration with writing had been replaced by a sense of competence: *My brain is always ready in here... Now I can actually write without getting all mad and sitting there doing nothing. Last year I could only write a bit and now I can get two or three paragraphs down... I like writing a lot more now and since I like it, I don't get frustrated when something happens... I like to write. I'm actually thinking about writing a small book...*

4. The intensive small group helped with auditory comprehension: *Half the time I don't get what my teacher says in class. But in here I can figure it out.*

5. The focus on content placed learning the skills of editing within the frame of the story: *Now that we don't worry about spelling I feel like we work on my ideas and I feel like a better writer... I have been working on my descriptive word choice...*

6. The reading/writing connection took on the shape of an upward spiral: *I have worked on using big words in my writing and then I learn to read it and I recognize that word later...*

Inside the alchemical container of this classroom, a new self-definition had emerged for the participants. When I asked Andrea Slocombe for her perspective on what it was about the program that had effected such wide-reaching change over such a short time, she replied that the sense of belonging arising from the personal welcome, the kinaesthetic work in the sand, the focus on oral language, and the focus on meaning in the writing all worked together to make the workshop effective. Andrea saw that, above all, the students had an imperative need to make accelerated progress in the area of oral language. The storymaking equipped them with skills in organizing, sequencing, and stating cause and effect, thereby giving them tools to explain what they were thinking in the classroom and in everyday conversation. Second, Andrea noted that becoming conversant with the technology was important. It meant that the boys were able to express their thoughts fully and independently without need for a scribe and without limiting their word choice to what they could write and spell. Independence with writing came with daily practice of recording meaningful stories using assistive devices of technology.

### *Example of growth over time*

The writing sample of one Grade 5 (age ten) student written within a time frame of 40 minutes on the first day of the workshop reads: 'There once was a peaceful little village called anamonwa the village anamois.'

Four months later, one school semester into the program, the same student wrote a second on-demand story within the identical time frame of 40 minutes. As you read it, notice that, in addition to the vast increase in the volume of writing, there is the building of suspense, the use of dialogue, and the navigation of different settings and points of view.

---

UNTITLED

One dark and rainy summer night there was a fire fighter who was coming home from a fire on 20 cardinal street. The fire was caused by a meteor that hit a house.

***

'Oh I hope mike gets home safely.' Lisa said with hope

'mom, David just broke my doll,' Carly blurted out through the silence of the night.

'David, stop that, and Carly stop being a tattletale, Lisa said annoyed.

'I'm not being a tatteltale'. Calry whined.

'Yes, you are, David said in a mocking voice.

'David htat's it. go to your room, and LArly to your,' Lisa said ferociously

'FINE!' david and Carly screamed.

They wander off mumbling angrily there fists quenched together tight. 'That's much better know I can cook dinner in peace.' There's a long moment of silence until, KABOOM CRACH BANG! 'You two keep it down up there.' KABOOM! 'That's it I'm comng up there' ...she found the kids crying in the cornere of the hallway. 'Are you kids okay?'

'Yyesd, ddad' carly managed to mumble before she started crying, Ok let's go doen stairs before the roof collapses. Crash just as the family kame down stairs the roof gv in to the blundering rain. 'you kids stay here I'm going to wait for your dad outside'

'Don't go mommy, I'm scared.

'I'll be right outside if you need me.'

## CONCLUSION

Centuries ago, the ancients posited two rhetorical categories: the *modus inveniendi* – the finding or discovery of arguments – and the *modus proferendi* – the presentation of those arguments in a persuasive way.[1] 'Find your ideas in the sand,' we tell the children. 'Then tell us the story.' We learn again what the ancients knew – discover, then express. This is the blueprint for the sandtray workshop. A foundational pattern.

Although the use of sandtray play for the teaching of language and literacy skills was born from the singular context of a Grade 2 (age seven) class challenged by multiple difficulties, the wide range of examples from this chapter shows the flexibility of the technique. Because it teaches a variety of academic, social, and emotional skills, it may be used to address the needs of students of many ages and competencies. My hope is that you will discover how to adapt its structures and possibilities to your own situation.

1 See, for example, St. Augustine's fourth-century treatise, *On Christian Teaching* (1995), where he takes up these categories, which, from his position as a teacher of rhetoric, he knew as the means for structuring his work. Books 1–3 detail the discovery of what must be learned, and Book 4 details the kind of eloquence required for presenting that learning.

# REFERENCES


Allan, J. and Bertoia, J. (1992) *Written Paths to Healing: Education and Jungian Child Counselling.* Dallas, TX: Spring Publications.

Allan, J. and Brown, K. (1993) 'Jungian play therapy in elementary schools.' *Elementary School Guidance and Counseling 28*, 1, 30–41.

Ashton-Warner, S. (1980) *Spinster.* London: Virago.

Ashton-Warner, S. (1963) *Teacher.* New York, NY: Simon and Schuster.

Atwell, N. (2002) *Lessons that Change Writers.* Portsmouth, ME: Heinemann.

Augustine (1995) *De Doctrina Christiana.* Translated and edited by R.P.H. Green. Oxford: Clarendon Press.

Barth, K. (1978) 'Mozart and the Negative Side of the Good Creation.' In J. McTavish and H. Wells (eds) *Preaching through the Christian Year.* Edinburgh: T&T Clark.

Beers, K. (2003) *When Kids Can't Read: What Teachers Can Do. A Guide for Teachers K–12.* Portsmouth, NH: Heinemann.

Bettelheim, B. (1977) *The Uses of Enchantment: The Meaning and Importance of Fairy Tales.* New York, NY: Vintage Books.

Bodger, J. (2000) *The Crack in the Teacup.* Toronto, ON: McClelland and Stewart.

Bodine, R.J. and Crawford, D. (1998) *The Handbook of Conflict Resolution Education: A Guide to Building Quality Programs in Schools.* San Francisco, CA: Jossey-Bass.

Booth, D. (2009) *Whatever Happened to Language Arts?* Markham, ON: Pembroke.

Bowlby, J. (1988) *Parent–Child Attachment and Healthy Human Development.* London: Routledge.

Bradway, K. (2006) 'What is sandplay?' *Journal of Sandplay Therapy 15*, 2, 7–9.

Bradway, K., Signell, K., Spare, G., Stewart, D., Stewart, L., and Thompson, C. (eds) (1990) *Sandplay Studies: Origins, Theory and Practice.* Boston, MA: Sigo Press.

Bruner, J.S. (1966) *Toward a Theory of Instruction.* Cambridge, MA: Harvard University Press.

Calkins, L. (2003) *Units of Study for Primary Writing: A Yearlong Curriculum.* New York, NY: Heinemann.

Calkins, L. and Mermelstein, L. (2003) *Launching the Writing Workshop.* New York, NY: Heinemann.

Calkins, L. and Oxenhorn, A. (2003) *Small Moments: Personal Narrative Writing.* New York, NY: Heinemann.

Cefai, C. and Cooper, P. (eds) (2009) *Promoting Emotional Education: Engaging Children and Young People with Social, Emotional and Behavioural Difficulties.* London: Jessica Kingsley Publishers.

Character Education Partnership (2008) *Performance Values: Why They Matter and What Schools Can Do to Foster Their Development. A Position Paper of the Character Education Partnership.* Washington, DC: Character Education Partnership. Available at www.drake.edu/icd/PDFs/Performance_Values.pdf, accessed on April 17, 2012.

Clarke, J.I. (1978) *Self-Esteem: A Family Affair.* Minneapolis, MN: Winston Press.

Clarke, J.I. and Dawson, C. (1998) *Growing Up Again: Parenting Ourselves, Parenting Our Children* (Second Edition). Center City, MN: Hazelden.

Colorosa, B. (2002) *Kids Are Worth It! Giving Your Child the Gift of Inner Discipline.* New York, NY: HarperCollins.

Cozolino, L. (2006) *The Neuroscience of Human Relationships: Attachment and the Developing Social Brain.* New York, NY: W.W. Norton.

Damasio, A.R. (1999) *The Feeling of What Happens: Body and Emotion in the Making of Consciousness.* New York, NY: Harcourt Brace.

Dennison, P. and Dennison, G. (1986) *Brain Gym: Simple Activities for Whole Brain Learning.* Ventura, CA: Edu-Kinesthetic, Inc.

Dorfman, L.R. and Capelli, R. (2007) *Mentor Texts.* Portland, ME: Stenhouse.

Douglas, C. (1993) *Translate This Darkness.* Princeton, NJ: Princeton University Press.

Dreikurs, R. (1964) *Children: The Challenge.* New York, NY: Penguin.

Durlak, J., Weissberg, R., Dymnicki, A., Taylor, R., and Schellinger, K. (2011) 'The impact of enhancing students' social and emotional learning: A meta-analysis of school-based universal interventions.' *Child Development, Special Issue: Raising Healthy Children, 82,* 1, 405–32.

Erikson, E. (1963) *Childhood and Society* (Second Edition). New York, NY: W.W. Norton.

Erikson, E. (1968) *Identity, Youth and Crisis.* New York, NY: W.W. Norton.

Escobedo, J. (2006) *Classroom Sandtray Storytelling and the Power of Play.* Paper presented at the 23rd Annual Association for Play Therapy International Conference, Toronto, ON.

Fletcher, R. (2006) *Boy Writers: Reclaiming Their Voices.* Portland, ME: Stenhouse/ Markham, ON: Pembroke.

Froebel, F. (2005) *The Education of Man.* New York, NY: Dover Publications. Originally published 1826.

Fulford, R. (1999) *The Triumph of Narrative: Storytelling in the Age of Mass Culture.* Toronto, ON: House of Anansi Press.

Goddard, H.C. (1956) *Blake's Fourfold Vision.* Wallingford, PA: Pendle Hill.

Goleman, D. (1998) *Working with Emotional Intelligence.* New York, NY: Bantam Books.

Gordon, T. (1977) *Leader Effectiveness Training.* New York, NY: Wyden Books.

Gravett, E. (2007) *Meerkat Mail.* New York, NY: Simon and Schuster.

*The Holy Bible. New Revised Standard Version* (1989). Nashville, TN: Thomas Nelson Publishers.

Hudson, J. and Shapiro, L. (1991) 'From Knowing to Telling: The Development of Children's Scripts, Stories, and Personal Narratives.' In A. McCabe and C. Peterson (eds) *Developing Narrative Structure.* Hillsdale, NJ: Erlbaum.

Huizinga, J. (1955) *Homo Ludens.* Boston, MA: Beacon Press.

Intini, J. (2010) 'Are we raising our boys to be underachieving men? The social and economic consequences of letting boys fall behind.' *Macleans,* October 18, 2010. Available at www2.macleans.ca/2010/10/18/raising-our-boys, accessed on February 6, 2012.

Jalongo, M.R. (2010) 'Listening in early childhood: An interdisciplinary review of the literature.' *International Journal of Listening 24,* 1, 1–18.

Jones, D. (2007) 'Speaking, listening, planning and assessing: The teacher's role in developing metacognitive awareness.' *Early Child Development and Care 177,* 6, 569–79.

Jung, C.G. (1965) *Memories, Dreams, Reflections* (Revised Edition). Translated by R. Winston and C. Winston. New York, NY: Vintage Books.

Jung, C.G. (1969) *Collected Works, Volume 8: The Structure and Dynamics of the Psyche* (Second Edition). Translated by R.F.C. Hull. Princeton, NJ: Princeton University Press.

Justice, L., Bowles, R., Kaderavek, J., Ukrainetz, T., Eisenberg, S., and Gillam, R. (2006) 'The index of narrative microstructure: A clinical tool for analyzing school-age children's narrative performances.' *American Journal of Speech-Language Pathology 15,* 2, 177–91.

Kaderavak, J. and Sulzby, E. (2000) 'Narrative production by children with and without specific language impairment: Oral narratives and emergent readings.' *Journal of Speech, Language and Hearing Research 43,* 34–49.

Kalff, D. (1980) *Sandplay: A Psychotherapeutic Approach to the Psyche.* Boston, MA: Sigo Press.

Kessler, R. (2000) *The Soul of Education.* Alexandria, VA: Association for Supervision and Curriculum Development.

Kestly, T. (2010) 'Group Sandplay in Elementary Schools.' In A.A. Drewes and C.E. Schaefer (eds) *School-Based Play Therapy* (Second Edition). Hoboken, NJ: John Wiley and Sons.

Krashen, S.D. (2003) *Explorations in Language Acquisition and Use: The Taipei Lectures.* Portsmouth, NH: Heinemann.

Landreth, G.L. (1993) 'Child-centred play therapy.' *Elementary School Guidance and Counselling 28,* 1, 17–29.

L'Engle, M. (1980) *Walking on Water.* Wheaton, IL: Harold Shaw.

Levin, P. (1988) *Becoming the Way We Are.* Deerfield Beach, FL: Health Communications.

Levitin, D.J. (2006) *This Is Your Brain on Music: The Science of a Human Obsession.* New York, NY: Penguin.

Lewis, C.S. (2005) 'The Weight of Glory.' In *Made for Heaven* New York, NY: HarperSanFrancisco.

Miller, C. and Boe, J. (1990) 'Tears into diamonds: Transformation of child psychic trauma through sandplay and storytelling.' *The Arts in Psychotherapy 17*, 3, 247–57.

Mitchell, R. and Friedman, H. (1994) *Sandplay: Past, Present and Future.* New York, NY: Routledge.

Neumann, E. (1988) *The Child: Structure and Dynamics of the Nascent Personality.* London: Maresfield Library.

Nicolopoulou, A., McDowell, J., and Brockmeyer, C. (2006) 'Narrative Play and Emergent Literacy: Storytelling and Story-Acting Meet Journal Writing.' In D.G. Singer, R.M. Golinkoff, and K. Hirsh-Pasek (eds) *Play = Learning: How Play Motivates and Enhances Children's Cognitive and Social-Emotional Growth.* Oxford: Oxford University Press.

Noddings, N. (1992) *Challenge to Care in Schools: An Alternative Approach to Education.* New York, NY: Teachers College Press, Columbia University.

Oliver, M. (1992) 'When Death Comes.' In *New and Selected Poems Volume One.* Boston, MA: Beacon Press.

Ontario Ministry of Education (2010) *Growing Success: Assessment, Evaluation, and Reporting in Ontario Schools. Covering Grades 1 to 12* (First Edition). Toronto, ON: Ministry of Education.

Piaget, J. (1923/1977) 'The Language and Thought of the Child.' In H. Gruber and J. Jacques Voneche (eds) *The Essential Piaget: An Interpretative Reference and Guide.* New York, NY: Basic Books.

Pochmursky, C. (Director) (2009) *The Musical Brain* (documentary motion picture). Canada: Matter of Fact Media in association with CTV and National Geographic Channels International. Originally aired January 31, 2009. Available at http://watch.ctv.ca/news/w-five/w-five-presents-the-musical-brain/#clip135235, accessed on Apil 17, 2012.

Pollack, W. (1998) *Real Boys: Rescuing Our Sons from the Myths of Boyhood.* New York, NY: Random House.

Rubin, P. (2001) 'Group Theraplay.' In A. Jernberg and P. Booth (eds) *Theraplay* (Second Edition). San Fransisco, CA: Jossey-Bass.

Rumi (1995) 'Send the Chaperones Away.' In *The Essential Rumi.* Translated by C. Barks. New York, NY: HarperSanFrancisco.

Rosenberg, M.B. (1999) *Nonviolent Communication: A Language of Compassion.* Del Mar, CA: Puddle Dancer Press.

Schore, A.N. (2000) 'Attachment and the regulation of the right brain.' *Attachment and Human Development 2*, 1, 23–47.

Schore, A.N. (2009) 'Right-Brain Affect Regulation: An Essential Mechanism of Development. Trauma, Dissociation, and Psychotherapy.' In D. Fossa, D. Siegel, and M. Solomon (eds) *The Healing Power of Emotion: Affective NeuroScience, Development and Clinical Practice.* New York, NY: W.W. Norton and Company.

Siegel, D. (2001) *Mindsight: The New Science of Personal Transformation.* New York, NY: Bantam Books.

Singer, D.G., Golinkoff, R.M., and Hirsh-Pasek, K (eds) (2006) *Play = Learning: How Play Motivates and Enhances Children's Cognitive and Social-Emotional Growth.* Oxford: Oxford University Press.

Stadler, M. and Ward, G.C. (2005) 'Supporting the narrative development of young children.' *Early Childhood Education Journal 33,* 2, 73–80.

Steig, W. (1969) *Sylvester and the Magic Pebble.* New York, NY: Simon and Schuster.

Stewart, L.H. (1990) 'Play and Sandplay.' In K. Bradway, K. Signell, G. Spare, D. Stewart, L. Stewart, and C. Thompson (eds) *Sandplay Studies: Origins, Theory and Practice.* Boston, MA: Sigo Press.

Tanner, L.N. (1997) *Dewey's Laboratory School: Lessons for Today.* New York, NY: Teachers College Press, Columbia University.

Tolkien, J.R.R. (1964) 'On Fairy-stories.' In *Tree and Leaf.* London: Unwin Books.

Tolkien, J.R.R. (1986) *The Hobbit.* New York, NY: Ballantine.

Vygotsky, L.S. (1986) *Thought and Language* (Revised Edition). Edited by A. Kozulin. Cambridge, MA: MIT Press. Originally published 1934.

Weil, S. (1987) 'The Symposium of Plato.' In *Intimations of Christianity among the Ancient Greeks.* London and New York, NY: Ark Paperbacks.

Weil, S. (1951) *Waiting for God.* New York, NY: Harper and Row.

Weinberg, B. (2007) 'Sandplay, the Psyche, and the Brain: What Is Happening Here?' In B. Weinberg and N. Baum (eds) *Sandplay and the Psyche: Inner Landscapes and Outer Realities.* Toronto, ON: Thera Art.

Weinrib, E.L. (1983) *Images of the Self.* Boston, MA: Sigo Press.

Wells, G. (1986) *The Meaning Makers: Children Learning Language and Using Language to Learn.* Portsmouth, NH: Heinemann.

Wells, H.G. (2005) *Little Wars and Floor Games (A Companion Piece to 'Little Wars').* Cirencester: The Echo Library. Originally published 1911.

Yeats, W.B. (1996) 'A Prayer for Old Age.' In R. Finneran (ed.) *The Collected Poems of W.B. Yeats* (Revised Second Edition). New York, NY: Simon and Schuster.

Zeman, L. (1995) *Gilgamesh the King (The Gilgamesh Trilogy).* Toronto, ON: Tundra Books.

Zimmer, H. (1971) *The King and the Corpse.* Edited by J. Campbell. Princeton, NJ: Bollingen Series XI, Princeton University Press.

# SUBJECT INDEX

# AUTHOR INDEX